The Social Construction of Mental Illness and Its Implications for Neuroplasticity

The Social Construction of Mental Illness and Its Implications for Neuroplasticity

Michael T. Walker

LEXINGTON BOOKS
Lanham • Boulder • New York • London

Published by Lexington Books
An imprint of The Rowman & Littlefield Publishing Group, Inc.
4501 Forbes Boulevard, Suite 200, Lanham, Maryland 20706
www.rowman.com

Unit A, Whitacre Mews, 26-34 Stannary Street, London SE11 4AB

This books is for educational purposes only and is not intended to be a substitute for the medical advice of a licensed physician. The reader should consult with their doctor in any matters relating to his/her mental health or health in general.

British Library Cataloguing in Publication Information Available

Library of Congress Cataloging-in-Publication Data

Names: Walker, Michael T., author.
Title: The social construction of mental illness and its implications for neuroplasticity / Michael T. Walker.
Description: Lanham : Lexington Books, [2016] | Includes bibliographical references and index.
Identifiers: LCCN 2016027460 (print) | LCCN 2016028075 (ebook) | ISBN 9781498524834 (cloth : alk. paper) | ISBN 9781498524841 (electronic)
Subjects: LCSH: Mental illness—Public opinion. | Mental illness—Social aspects. | Neuroplasticity.
Classification: LCC RC455.2.P85 W35 2016 (print) | LCC RC455.2.P85 (ebook) | DDC 305.9/084--dc23
LC record available at https://lccn.loc.gov/2016027460

™ The paper used in this publication meets the minimum requirements of American National Standard for Information Sciences Permanence of Paper for Printed Library Materials, ANSI/NISO Z39.48-1992.

Printed in the United States of America

Contents

Preface

When I say "mental illness" is a social construction, I'm not saying people aren't suffering. Yes, human beings experience deep and prolonged subjective distress often accompanied by great performative difficulties that take tremendous tolls on their lives and the lives of their loved ones. At the effect of dominating perceptions we can be paralyzed into inaction or propelled impulsively into acting against our better judgment and long-term interests. A person's subjectivity can be so lopsidedly subjective that they're effectively "buried in their head" and as a result their preoccupation with their inner world is at the expense of their outer world (e.g., social) competency. Our lives can be impoverished by rigid negative beliefs and circumscribed by countless fears. To make matters worse, self-deception is the rule, not the exception. This is the human condition.

Some human difficulties are easy to not label as illnesses. Stress over a job situation or relationship are included here. But what about the extreme examples? What about people who hear people talking in their heads, or have uncontrollable excitement leading to uncontrollable impulsive behavior, or people paralyzed by fear, or people who just seem to inhabit a world far from the consensual one, or others hell-bent, without conscience, on hurting or destroying other people? Surely this is a medical illness. Isn't it? Something must be broken!

We have been trained to think and perceive like this. The institutions of reductionist science, medicine, and psychology have conditioned our minds to think like this; and as a result a particular "clinical" world appears as "obvious" and "objective." While at the gym, we see a person wearing a red cape, full of energy, talking very fast while arguing with someone and our very next thought is "this person is 'bipolar.'" Yet "bipolar" is not a category in nature, it's a label, an abstraction. The behaviors and subjective experience are real; the abstraction (label) is definitely optional.

We all live on a *continuum* of human developmental transformation and at some point on this *continuum* we realize our fundamental human equality and solidarity that comes with the recognition of our common subjective dilemma. In other words, part of our maturation as human beings involves recognizing that each of us experiences our world as if we had direct and unmediated access to the world *as it is*, as opposed to as it appears. People often realize this on some superficial level ("I realize this is my perspective"); but where this affects our lives the most is at the level of culturally and institutionally transmitted fundamental and hidden assumptions about what it means to be human. Notions of normality/abnormality and "mental illness" hide us from this subjective dilemma and fundamental equality—the pot is forever calling the kettle black. Making comparisons in our egoism—as to who's better and who's worse—short-circuits our transformative efforts. Similarly with the clinical reality in the mental health profession and its illusion of objectivity. We will see that this illusion of objectivity profoundly impairs our ability to facilitate change in our clients.

It would take the postmodern worldview to recognize how the realities we inhabit don't exist independent of their human occupants, but are socially constructed in language. Ernst Cassirer (1963) pointed out that we don't even have pure sense perception to begin with; in other words, what we sense (e.g., with our eyes and ears) is already a product of interpretation. This order or construction imposed on our experience of people is purely a result of sentences and conversations that *presume* the existence of clinical categories. To discuss to what degree "schizophrenia" has a genetic component is to reaffirm the supposition that "schizophrenia" exists independently of the behaviors and subjective experiences that it is operationally defined by—that it exists like a broken bone exists. This is just like when the ancient Greeks presupposed the existence of Ares and Aphrodite when they argued whether the two were lovers or not—*reality-creating suppositions are embedded in sentences*. The gods were real as long as they were spoken into existence.

Because of this assumed and taken-for-granted clinical reality we simply don't recognize the profound disabling effects of this way of constructing (interpreting) human beings. Or, at best, because the clinical world seems objective (reflecting reification and an unwarranted link to scientific legitimacy) we might think these effects, though unfortunate, inevitable. The antistigma campaign is only a superficial attempt to address this problem without addressing the real issue. This is true for all the Diagnostic and Statistical Manual (DSM)/International Statistical Classification of Diseases (ICD) categories, from post-traumatic stress disorder (PTSD), to schizophrenia, to depression, to bipolar, to panic attacks, to hording, to obsessive-compulsive disorder (OCD), to attention deficit/hyperactivity disorder (ADHD)—just to mention a few of the trendy ones. If we stop manufacturing "mental illness" we don't need to fight stigma.

The intransigence of counterproductive behavior and subjective experience are not proof of "illness." With our new knowledge of complexity neuroscience and neuroplasticity we know that behavior patterns (and their associated mental and emotional states) have *neurocorrelates* and in the adult human brain neural circuits are a kind of wiring that doesn't change so easily, *but they do change*. As we'll see, *repetitive* changes in behavior, thinking, and language alter the physical structure of the brain.

But in order for this to happen we have to have the right paradigm, worldview, context, perspective, vocabulary—and the current one of psychiatric diagnoses is not only *not* supporting neuroplasticity, it is preventing it! Amazingly and ironically, as we will see, this is true of the well-intentioned leaders of the neuroplasticity and mindfulness movements. Though they proclaim the brain's malleability and the life changing efficacy of mindfulness, in those same sentences they use words like "patient," "depression," and "treatment"—all the lexicon of the clinical worldview. (Note, this is not a matter of political correctness, it's a matter of two different realities, two different universes of possibilities. "Political correctness" is what happens when you introduce a new vocabulary without providing the context that supports it.) The pragmatic impulse of mental health has bumped up against a roof from which it can be liberated only by way of postmodernism and its linguistic paradigm.

Another reason people cling to the disease interpretation is genetic correlations and the artificial/false dichotomy of nature versus nurture. Any biological/genetic aspect of behavior or personality must mean it's a disease. It's often naively assumed that mental issues are *either* a result of our genetics *or* our childhood experiences. Though the dichotomy is a false one to begin with, the controversy itself implies genetic determinism: genes = destiny. As we will discuss later, when you're operating with false assumptions what's implicit and connotative (context) is more important to examine than what's explicit and denotative (content).

Biological or genetic correlations are not proof of "illness"—our genes are not our destiny. Genetics and experience are inextricably intertwined. Bruce Lipton demonstrates in his *Biology of Belief* (2008) how much power our environment, actions, lifestyles, beliefs, and feelings alter the expression of our genes—this is the field of *epigenetics*. When it comes to our bodies, our lifestyle and environment feed back into our DNA in such a way as to alter its expression; for example, exercise and nutrition avoid or reduce the expression of the genetic propensity for many physical diseases. Diabetes—the once cherished companion analogy to the "chemical imbalance"—is often used to make the analogy between insulin and psychiatric medications in terms of being "in balance" and living a "normal" life. As it turns out diabetes is very controllable with diet and exercise (Campbell and Campbell, 2006)—many people with diabetes get off their medications. So much for the old beloved analogy.

When we're talking about the human brain, infinitely more malleable than our pancreas, the "disease" metaphor is far more inadequate. With the right training the brain can alter or override both its genetic and conditioned (or learned) propensities. The key word being *propensities*. As we'll see in our discussion of complex systems (of which the human brain is a prime example), emergent properties (e.g., thinking, language) feedback and alter or temper the expression of lower level operations (e.g., genetics or conditioning). In other words, the brain takes itself on, thus altering its otherwise default neuronal and genetic expression; and psychotherapy is the catalyst to this process. Richard Glass (2008), *noted researcher in evidence-based medicine* at the University of Chicago, summarizes the new consensus:

> Recent research in brain imaging, molecular biology, and neurogenetics has shown that psychotherapy changes brain function and structure. Such studies have shown that psychotherapy affects regional cerebral blood flow, neurotransmitter metabolism, gene expression, and persistent modifications in synaptic plasticity. (1589)

Yes, gene expression!

So the brain's genetic propensities and expression are altered on *two* levels: (1) at the level of DNA expression—in other words, at the same level that the rest of the body benefits from a healthy diet, exercise, nurturing circumstances, and emotional well-being—and (2) at the level of neuroplasticity, where the brain transcends itself. Interestingly, as we will see, changes in thinking, feeling, and behavior alter both the neuronal circuitry of the brain (i.e., neuroplasticity) *and* the genetic expression of the brain (epigenetics). In an attempt at scientific objectivity (with the use of statistics; the Diagnostic and *Statistical* Manual—DSM) the mental health profession *labels* what would otherwise be called propensities or habits, thereby locking them in.

Like the lifestyle changes to cure diabetes, altering the physical structure of our brain through repetitive practice in both language, perspective, and action—thereby feeling and performing better in the various arenas in our lives—is hard work. However, the "patient" identity manufactured in the mental health profession (chapter 9) is nowhere near up to this. By and large, the "patient" is responsible only to make his/her appointments on time and take his/her medications as prescribed. Furthermore, the "patient's" *script* includes passivity, insecurity, avoidance, assumed incompetence, a lack of confidence, and a persistent preoccupation with the dreaded possibility of a recurrence of their "illness" (the assumption being that the best they can do is "live with their 'illness'").

As we'll discuss later in chapter 10 with the right vocabulary (words, perspectives, and practices) "the patient" is transformed into the artist, the writer, the painter, the musician, the cultural critic, the philosopher, the scientist, the entertainer, the therapist/coach, or the spiritual leader. If Virginia Wolfe were alive today—in today's clinical reality—she'd most likely be in a board and care, on supplemental security income (SSI), and preoccupied all day long with which one of her roommates stole her disabled bus pass (i.e., she'd be a "patient"). Creativity and imagination are the calling of the twenty-first century (chapter 10)!

This book results from the convergence of three crucial areas of practice and investigation: complexity neuroscience, psychotherapy outcome studies, and postmodern psychotherapy. Their conclusions are startlingly similar: psychotherapy is an art form based in a collaborative relationship founded upon empathy, non-judgmental relating, authenticity, attunement, feedback-informed dialogic responsiveness, therapist mindfulness, and tailor-made problem redescription. We will see that it is the language paradigm that will finally give us the required receptivity, presence, and interpretive flexibility to realize this way of being and helping.

Psychiatric diagnoses and their medical framework are the ultimate in restraining contexts when considering what works in psychotherapy. In today's modernist (in contrast to postmodernist) world psychiatric diagnoses and their clinical context appear as real as the chair you're sitting on. All attempts to be client driven, wellness focused, recovery oriented, solution focused, strength based, feedback informed, non-judgmentally observant, or accurately empathetic are *surface phenomena* layered on top of a bedrock of the clinical world. The clinical world is just the opposite: practitioner driven, illness focused, problem focused, deficit based, feedback immune, judgmentally observant, and inaccurately empathetic.

It would only be from a postmodern investigation outside of the mental health profession (e.g., in literature, history, and philosophy) that it becomes clear that the entire clinical worldview of the mental health profession, including the idea of "mental illness," is a construction in language, a vocabulary. The clinical vocabulary's (aka medical model's) pseudo-link with science does not exempt it from being a cultural artifact, i.e., being one vocabulary among others. Later we will further deconstruct the clinical vocabulary with an investigation into its historical origins.

There are many other reasons why people zealously embrace the disease model in mental health and in addiction treatment. Among the reasons is a feeling of helplessness. The medical model has made professionals and public alike quick to label and very slow at developing the interpersonal perspective and skill required to support another fellow human being struggling with the complexity of the human condition and that of the modern world. Said another way, the medicalization of problems in living has as a whole made the entire profession "dependent on medications," which has made its practitioners deficient in the skills needed to produce lasting change. Society as a whole resorts to labeling in the face of its own intolerance of individual uniqueness and its inadequate skills in inspiring others and holding them accountable when appropriate. In the face of helplessness people label. The mental health profession has not tapped into the power of language and neuroplasticity.

Don't confuse correlation with causation! Everyone knows the brain is involved in behavior/thinking/feeling. What's not so well known is that changes in behavior/thinking/feeling—when done repetitively—change the brain. In light of the discovery of neuroplasticity, we are not determined by our childhood conditioning, nor are we genetically determined, but we need a radical change in perspective to take advantage of these facts. As we will see, mindfulness and repetitive changes in our thinking, language, perspective, and behavior alter the physical structure of the human brain. Neural *correlation* has been confused by medicalization (the illness model) as one-way neuro*causation*. Causation goes both ways and the term "correlation" works better in terms of implying this; or we can say that the brain and behavior/thinking/language are *reflexively* or *recursively* related.

I use the terms "reflexivity" (e.g., reflexively related) or "recursiveness" (e.g., recursively related) throughout the book to describe how two things in a relationship sequentially influence each other in a feedback loop. A influences B, then B_2 (changed B) feeds back and influences A, then A_2 (changed A) influences B_2—back and forth ad infinitum. For example, thinking influences action, the results of which feed back into the thinking, which then results in a new action. The phenomenon of reflexivity (recursiveness) may be an indication of the fundamental unity and interconnectedness of all things.

I believe the mental health profession to be largely ignorant of the implications of neuroplasticity for practice, training, and research. One exception is Allan Schore (2012), a leading researcher and practitioner in interpersonal neurobiology:

> We are now faced with the problem of how this rapidly expanding body of discoveries in development and neuroscience will be used in the mental health professions, not only in the delivery of service but also in the training of the next generation of psychotherapists. Older ideas about what is required for a basic knowledge base for all health care professionals must now be updated and radically altered. (9)

Currently in the small circles where neuroplasticity is the operating principle, I believe its practical implications to be in their infancy. The neuroscientists' redescribing difficulties with thinking, feeling, and behavior as the overworking or underworking of various brain structures is a good beginning but hardly sufficient. Likewise nor does mindfulness practice suffice, by itself, on the difficult and changing playing field of life. Schore's right brain (i.e., emotional and unconscious) and interpersonal revolution has opened up the domains of subjectivity and intersubjectivity, respectively—a breakthrough indeed, but just a beginning. This book is a critical contribution to this call for a radically altered profession.

I'm not writing primarily to advocate a particular kind of approach to helping people. I'm here to open up the field, to free it from the ice age of dead metaphors, categorical imperatives (not Kantian meaning), and institutional trance. The profession's medical worldview as absolute/objective truth is the problem, not the time-tested dialogic skills and perspectives of its agents (practitioners). I'm not antipsychiatry. Nor do I believe the mental health profession to be solely an expression of the will to power or social control (Michel Foucault). And, of course, no sensible person could deny that people have serious subjective and performative difficulties (a mistaken criticism based on a misinterpretation of what Thomas Szasz [1961] meant by "myth of mental illness"). These critical perspectives form only part of the whole picture that reveals psychotherapy to be a dialogic art form.

Fifty-five years have passed since Thomas Szasz wrote *The Myth of Mental Illness*. He never denied that people had serious emotional difficulties and problems living as his detractors often accused him of. He believed that it was entirely arbitrary and a mistake to call this a "mental illness," and that doing so resulted in a disabling identity and social ostracism. He asserted that *all people* needed help living responsible and moral lives. He recognized the power of language. Yet, 1960s America was not ready to hear his postmodern message. Today's advances in neuroscience, outcome studies, and postmodern therapies have provided the needed context for Szasz. Szasz helped construct the necessary context that will finally liberate us to far more effectively and efficiently realize what works in psychotherapy—psychotherapy as an art form.

James Bugental's *The Art of the Psychotherapist: How to Develop the Skills That Take Psychotherapy beyond Science* (1987) and Allan Schore's *The Science of the Art of Psychotherapy* (2012) were prototypes of this work. And, of course, I'd be remiss without acknowledging the consummate artist of intersubjectivity, Carl Rogers. I reference Rogers a lot not because I'm a proponent of client-centered therapy but because his relational stance and core therapeutic conditions (unconditional positive regard, accurate empathy, and therapist congruence or authenticity) are a theme repeated over and over again (explicitly or implicitly) in the cutting-edge areas of investigation of psychotherapy: interpersonal neurobiology, psychotherapeutic outcome studies, and postmodern psychotherapy. What is meant by the art of psychotherapy will be a major topic of this book.

The dynamic dialogic connection with people, the subtleties of language and non-verbal responses, the right brain to right brain resonance, the experimentation with redescription all require a here-and-now receptivity, presence, and flexibility of responsiveness that characterizes an art form. This dialogic connection along with non-judgmental relating, deep empathy, and authenticity creates what's now being called *intersubjectivity*, the intersubjective field, or intersubjective space (characterized by attunement and resonance); and it is intersubjectivity that is the crucible within which human transformation takes place. As we will see the clinical metaphor with its rigid categories and prescribed roles all but blinds us to the nuances and subtleties required to co-create and maintain intersubjective space as well as to formulate new problem/solution descriptions that resonate with people and empower them *to choose* in accordance with their commitment to the quality of their lives. Furthermore, the transformation of the profession and its training will benefit all the human services and the public as a whole.

Finally, as health care reform moves us in the direction of prevention, efficiency, effectiveness, and accountability we can no longer afford to be bound by time-honored assumptions, categories, and theories. This book represents a coherent framework allowing us to make the transition from a *theoretical orientation* to a *practical orientation* in a way that's consistent with the new frontier of complexity neuroscience.

A NOTE TO THE ACADEMICALLY MINDED

The difficulty in writing this book is that the book represents the paradigm shift in mental health from being an aspiring-to-be science to an art. The writing of an academic book takes place within in the scientific/academic paradigm which demands factual and logical rigor as well as being situated in the professional research literature. The writing of an academic book *about a new paradigm* still requires this logical rigor, only with data that doesn't cohere with the old paradigm. This book is about extending, interpreting, and drawing warranted conclusions about the current existing data that *contradicts* the prevailing clinical paradigm in mental health. In a sense, I'm "connecting the dots" that *don't fit into the old paradigm*; but as we will see, they form a striking new and profound pattern.

To complicate matters further, the logical rigor contained herein has revealed a new paradigm that has, in turn, led us *beyond theory* and into a conceptual framework whose sole purpose is to *support practice* and yet is still compatible with science—or at least complexity neuroscience. In this sense it is similar to James Prochaska and Carlo DiClemente's (1983) and Prochaska, DiClemente, and John Norcross's (1992) Transtheoretical Model. Furthermore, I will argue that complexity neuroscience—the human brain seen as a whole, as a complex system, in its social environment and with its adaptive capabilities—is *the* mental health profession's *legitimate tie* to scientific authority.

This book is an advancement in postmodern theory and practice in mental health; it is indeed a breakthrough in the postmodern approach. It is intended to reach the postmodern audience as well as those who are otherwise open-minded and committed to producing results in their work with people. This being the case, I have devoted the section "Paradigm Shifts and Incommensurability" in chapter 1 to address some concerns and considerations that could be leveled at what may look from the traditional paradigm to be a fairly polemical, unconventional, somewhat unacademic, and seemingly unempirical and biased work. So for those readers used to an academic framework and tone I recommend reading that section before continuing. For those readers unbothered by the content, style, and tone of this work so far I recommend skipping that section.

For anyone having difficulty with the recognition that language creates realities I recommend "The Paradox of Reality and Interpretation" in chapter 5.

IF YOU OR YOUR CLIENTS ARE TAKING PSYCHIATRIC MEDICATIONS NOW

Don't stop. Chances are you/they don't have the skills and perspectives to manage yourself/themselves sufficiently for all concerned. This is the current state of affairs of this medication-dependent society we live in. You don't stop using your crutch just because you've read a book about physical therapy that reveals to you that life without your crutch is *possible*. Moreover, it's been my experience that people who listen to me or read my material sometimes use it as an *excuse* to stop taking their "medications."

The current institutional, professional, and legal world—of which I'm a grateful member—requires that you always discuss getting off psychiatric medications with your doctor.

As will be discussed, the postmodern view of medications is that they are one tool among many in the herculean journey of recognizing, transcending, transforming, or otherwise coping with *the human condition*. I'm not *against* medications. I'm *for* what works. I'm *for* people becoming stronger human beings and therefore becoming less dependent on everything.

We don't have to "be a patient" (see chapter 9 on the creation of "the patient") or believe in the "chemical imbalance" idea to use psychiatric medications. Like every other substance we put in our bodies they have, *when used as recommended*, a discernable effect or not. A psychiatrist is a resource; pills are a tool. We want to experiment with different lifestyles, strategies, tools, skills, and perspectives in order to do more of what works and less of what doesn't work.

On the whole, I have nothing against psychiatric "medications"; I do have a problem with the "horror story" that they're embedded in: you have a "chemical imbalance," you have an illness (e.g., "bipolar disorder"), you have to take these medications the rest of your life, and if you get off your medications again you'll be back in the hospital and lose everything again. This book could have been subtitled "A New, Healthier Context for Psychiatric Medications."

AN APOLOGY IN ADVANCE

I would like to apologize in advance if anyone—professional, client, or layperson—is offended or insulted by my work. In my fervor to get this important and eminently humane message out, I may not always word things best or provide enough context. The text is sometimes polemical, sometimes hyperbolic, often informally written, and often poetic—as such exemplifying the way in which right brain to right brain (i.e., emotive) transformation happens (chapter 2).

Though at times it looks like I'm doing a demolition job, my intention always is to improve the profession by eliminating its weaknesses and building on its strengths. Furthermore, "the mental health profession" is an abstraction as well, composed of human beings just like myself; and like myself we're all thrown into a world and imprinted with its already always predicated ways of speaking and being—all of which represent a current historical moment of cultural evolution. We're all in the same dilemma of subjectivity. We're all standing on a mountain of those who have come before us and are to varying degrees limited in our access to the best human intelligence to date by no fault of our own. Moreover, the mental health profession is a subset of Western culture as a whole, and all my criticisms of the profession are criticisms of Western culture. Though I'm a critic of the profession, I love the profession as I recognize it as part of humanity's historical transcendent tradition. Lastly, please criticize me. Though I put my work out in a tone of conviction, I'm aware that there's plenty of room for dialogue and subsequent refinement and revision of my views. But more than critique, I would hope that in a spirit of a common commitment to the civilizing human enterprise we, like other artists in other historical periods, could work collaboratively and build upon each other's creativity.

Acknowledgments

I would like to thank my family and friends over the years that have encouraged me to write this book. Among other things, I'm grateful for my mother for her conventionality and my father for his unconventionality; I was fortunate enough to get enough of each to succeed in the institutional world without the sacrifice of my creativity.

I would like to thank Jennifer Andrews and David Clark for including me in their postmodern cabal at Phillips Graduate Institute in Encino, California, where in the 1990s I was exposed to the leaders of the postmodern psychotherapy movement. I'm grateful to Tom Grauman, whose unconventional and philosophical mind made us natural collaborators in Vancouver, British Columbia, in the summer of 2011. I want to thank Marilyn Jhung for being open to this work and taking the institutional baton from me. I would also like to extend my gratitude to all my clients over the past twenty-five years; without their participation I wouldn't have been able to develop this perspective and these practices—a special thanks to the people I worked with at "the red brick building."

I would also like to say how grateful I am to Tony Bevacqua for promoting my work and encouraging me to write this book. I'm indebted to John Travers for including me as a trainer in his "peer advocate" training program from which my ideas received invaluable feedback. I want to express my gratitude to Allen Francis for his brilliance of insight and boldness of action in his attempt to Save Normal. I'm also forever grateful for all the members of the mental health consumer movement in the United States, with whom I've felt a great sense of solidarity. I thank my editors at Lexington Books, Amy King and Kasey Beduhn, who provided valuable feedback and welcomed enthusiasm throughout the course of this journey.

I am indebted to the thinkers in literature, history, philosophy, science, and psychology I represent in this synthesis. I would like to thank Michael Thompson for being my friend and thinking partner. Finally, I especially would like to thank Arnold Siegel, whose coursework in Autonomy and Life has made a profound impact on my life, and as such has indirectly made this book possible.

Introduction

In our positivistic era, where all aspects of human life are seen as understandable, predicable, and controllable by way of reason and rationality, it is rare when science gives way to art. This is understandable, indeed, as reason and rationality were justifiably deified as they pulled us out of the Dark Ages and into the Enlightenment and the modern era. On the one hand science, technology, industry, and medicine brought us untold possibilities of relieving human suffering; on the other hand tolerance, liberal democracy, and enlightened economic policies brought forth a never before realized distribution of wealth.

In response to the relativism (Sophism) of his time, Plato asserted reason's dominance over poetry. Thus began the long hegemony of reason (e.g., philosophy) and science. The practical value and seeming endless applications of reason seemed to imply that all the mysteries of the universe and of ourselves would eventually come under its purview.

Ironically, toward the end of the twentieth century science finally met its limit when it turned its methods toward the human brain. Though the scientific legitimacy of psychiatry and psychology has long been questioned, the death knell of their conceptual foundations in science has sounded as neuroscience reaches some degree of maturity in the form of *complexity neuroscience*. Complexity neuroscience has established that our brains are not machines with occasional missing or broken parts.

The pliability of the human brain has been under our noses all the time; like Jonathan Swift's Laputins, it was only the spell of science, being bound and circumscribed by categories, that kept us from seeing it. Moreover as we will also see, what works in psychotherapy (e.g., relationship, engagement, alliance) has been painfully obvious as well, not to the therapist as "technician," but to the therapist as artist, often referred to as master therapists.

Swift's Laputins were a parody of what Martin Heidegger (1927/1962) called the *theoretical ontology*; in other words, a way of being anchored in the theoretically based categories of science or social science. We see through (only see) the abstractions (including their network of presuppositions) that science (or in our case social science) has come up with and sanctioned. The same is true with self-help categories and the stereotypes of "cultural competency." As Kevin Cope, a noted postmodern literary critic, puts it in his 1990 *Criteria of Certainty: Truth and Judgment in the English Enlightenment*: "Of all the lands that he portrays, Swift evidences the least sympathy for Laputa, where Cartesian thinking systematically conflicts with practice. 'I have not seen a more clumsy, awkward, and unhandy people'" (quoting *Gulliver's Travels*; 123). Cartesian thinking is reductive thinking (oversimplified, mistaking a part for the whole) and the mistake of applying reductive thinking to complex systems, namely human beings and the human brain, is a major theme of this book. This is in contrast to *having eyes that see* evidence of neuroplasticity everywhere as well as all the subtleties of relationship and communication (verbal, non-verbal, emotional) that empower.

But, again, ironically being led by the nose by reductive science—*reductive* neuroscience eventually yielding to *complexity* neuroscience—we discovered that the brain is not a machine, but instead was a complex system operating under the new rules of complexity science. The emergent properties of the brain allow for (1) higher (thinking) centers to transcend or temper the lower (feeling) centers and (2) more adaptive interpretive frames to subsume less adaptive ones. Counterproductive patterns of thinking, feeling, and behaving through relanguaging and training can be exchanged for more productive and satisfying ones.

Many neuroscientists soon became enamored with the relationship between the mind, the brain, and relationship. Soon they enumerated certain relationship qualities that were essential to facilitating brain integration and proper functioning; namely, unconditional positive regard, empathy, authenticity, attunement, and collaborative reinterpretation of client and his/her situation. Attachment theory became forever wedded to complexity neuroscience only to give birth to interpersonal neurobiology.

Interestingly, two other areas of professional inquiry converged and validated the conclusions of interpersonal neurobiology; these were the investigators doing psychotherapy outcome research and postmodern theorists and practitioners.

Additionally, the postmodernists claimed that "knowledge" is power and both are intrinsic in human relationships. In postmodern circles the understanding of the determinative power of language itself in human relationships began superficially and more in theory than practice. As part of this postmodern tradition, this book aims to bring the power of language to forefront not only in theory but also in practice—this is the language paradigm.

Another theme of this book is that the most obvious impediment to these proven relationship qualities is the clinical and institutional vocabulary. Far from being an absolute/objective reality, the clinical and institutional world is spoken into existence. Yes, what we call "mental illness" and all its "diagnoses" are social constructions. Having been thus constructed we see them everywhere. The illusion is that these categories exist in nature independent of human beings' comprehension and that we simply name them as they are discovered. When the truth is that they are statistically based abstractions unrelated to any common neuronal cause (a dolphin is not a fish)—unlike physical conditions. The question is how do these labels or categories square with the new knowledge of the brain, the conclusions of psychotherapy outcome research, and the perspectives and practices of postmodern therapy. Now we are finally in a position to evaluate the consequences of these vocabularies.

The point of this book is to make it clear that the idea of "mental illness" is a social construction; meaning the idea of mental illness—and all its subdivisions of psychiatric "diagnoses" (bipolar disorder, schizophrenia, post-traumatic stress disorder [PTSD], obsessive-compulsive disorder [OCD], depression)—are made up. They are words used to classify people according to similarities in behavior and subjective experience (thought and feeling).

The Diagnostic and Statistical Manual (DSM) was a rough-and-ready attempt at understanding human beings with difficulty with living. One can imagine, before all the sundry categories that exist today, that in an attempt to understand "abnormal" human behavior, psychiatry looked to statistically categorize the varieties of "abnormalities"—simply run statistical analyses on data, sort, content analysis, etc., until patterns or clusters emerge into the categories familiar today. Psychiatry, with its roots in medicine, obviously—linking brain to behavior—would view the external behavior as "symptoms" of internal biological "disease" in the brain. This is the historically and socially constructed lens (bias) with which the psychiatric profession began (and continues) to look at human behavior outside the norm. As we will discover, this one-way causal assumption will turn out to be not only wrong but to have devastating consequences.

Moreover, to say something is a social construction is to mean that in the course of cultural evolution (history) human beings make up words, metaphors, and concepts that create new perspectives and contexts to help us negotiate the environments in which we find ourselves. Even the meanings of existing words change to forward their practical value. The essential postmodern point is that language is a tool to help us in our practical living and not something that represents some essential "thing" that exists in the world independent of language (in philosophy known as the thing it itself—an entity absent any perceptual bias). This is especially true when we're talking about the human brain, subjective experience, and behavior. On the other hand, for practical purposes, we can obviously say that the word "chair" represents the "thing" we sit on.

Another way in which so-called "mental illness" is a social construction is the way in which the diagnostic categories and other professional language and practices are self-fulfilling. Once you call somebody "bipolar" they (and whoever else in their life that is privy to this assignment) view their lives and difficulties through this lens. You can no longer be excited or angry without being "manic." Your dreams, preferences, and concerns for your life are secondary (if that) to "stabilizing the condition." Ironically (as we'll see in chapter 13 on postmodern coaching) engaging people in their interests, passions, projects, and purposes provides the context and motivation with which to make better decisions, control unproductive behaviors, and to acquire a greater degree of personal responsibility.

Clinical language locks the person (aka patient) and his or her social network into a clinical, deficit-based, pathologized interpretation of his or her life. The "diagnosis" has everyone focusing on the "symptoms"—yes, believing is seeing. The French author Anaïs Nin (1961, 124) quotes the Jewish Talmud: "We don't see things as *they are,* we see things as *we are.*" Moreover, we know from common sense that the more you focus on something the more you get of it. This is what we call iatrogenic illness or "illness" incurred as a result of the "treatment."

We'll have more to say about social constructionism later, but for now we'll turn our attention to the focal point of the psychiatric vocabulary: the Diagnostic and Statistical Manual or DSM (1952, 1968, 1978, 1980, 1987, 1994, 2000, 2013). And, of course, everything I have to say about the DSM classification system holds true for the International Statistical Classification of Diseases (ICD; 1949–1992) classification system of "mental and behavioral disorders" (chapter 5, F00–F99). Both systems use "symptom" clusters and "functional impairment" to classify "mental disorders" and in most cases the definitions are the same. For example when switching from DSM to ICD when it comes to "major depression, recurrent with psychotic features" you simply change the numeric code from 296.34 to F33.3; this is the case for the vast majority of the psychiatric "disorders"—just changing the numeric code. There may be slight variations in definitions, but the principle of defining a "diagnosis" by "symptoms" is exactly the same. From this point on, for the sake of brevity and readability, I'll only mention the DSM, keeping in mind that it will always be assumed that what I'm saying holds identically true to the ICD.

The psychiatric bible, the DSM is a classification system (of psychiatric "diagnoses") based on statistics. Of course, we can look at thousands of people and see which sets of behaviors tend to go together and then give each set a label. Each "diagnosis" has its "criteria"; for example, "depression" is the label given when a person experiences daily five of the nine items below (not including #10, which is required for all psychiatric diagnoses):

1. Depressed mood or irritable most of the day, nearly every day, as indicated by either subjective report (e.g., feels sad or empty) or observation made by others (e.g., appears tearful)
2. Significant weight change (5 percent) or change in appetite
3. Decreased interest or pleasure in most activities, most of each day
4. Change in sleep: Insomnia or hypersomnia

5. Change in activity: Psychomotor agitation or retardation
6. Fatigue or loss of energy
7. Guilt/worthlessness: Feelings of worthlessness or excessive or inappropriate guilt
8. Concentration: Diminished ability to think or concentrate, or more indecisiveness
9. Suicidality
10. Functional impairment. This is a criterion for all psychiatric diagnoses. It is the way in which our current subjective state affects our daily living, relationships, work, etc.

These behaviors tend to go together (statistically) and are therefore given a name ("depression") to signify when five or more occur together. From this perspective the label simply refers to a set of subjective experiences and behaviors. In other words, the DSM (with its checklists) is like a field guide, much as a naturalist uses to identify birds or trees.

Since the field of clinical psychology and psychiatry are considered medical specialties they exist in a medical context of disease and illness. In this context these subjective states and observable behaviors are transformed into "symptoms" and the unobservable source of the symptoms is the "illness." The word "symptom" always implies a causal agent called a "disease." According to this *narrative*, the point is to correctly diagnose the cause of the "symptoms" in order to intervene with the right "treatment."

The labeling of "symptom" clusters as a "diagnosis" implies that there is an "illness" *causing* the "symptoms." The label or "diagnosis" no longer stands for a group of co-occurring subjective experiences and observable behaviors. In the medical context the label (or diagnosis) is the *cause* of the co-occurring states and behaviors (called "symptoms"). The problem, as we will see in chapter 7, is that—as the makers of the DSM readily admit—using the most sophisticated equipment available no identifiable and measurable "gene or neurotransmitter or circuitry explanation" (Frances, 2013a) for any of the "diagnoses" has ever been identified!

The crucial mistake is made when we call these behaviors and subjective experiences "symptoms" and the label designating a cluster of "symptoms" a "diagnosis." Up until this point we've just engaged in an interesting word game, sorting people into categories based on common behaviors and subjective experiences.

But once we use the terms "symptoms" and "diagnoses" we've just created a "patient" with a "mental illness" and a "diagnosis"—together with other interwoven concepts and practices (e.g., biopsychosocial assessment, resistance, compliance, case management, integrated care, medications, triage) we've created a clinical reality. Throughout the book I will use the terms "old paradigm," "clinical reality," "prevailing mental health paradigm," and "medical model" synonymously. Moreover, it is widely believed that the "diagnosis" is caused by a "chemical imbalance" (which, as we will see later, is a metaphor which doesn't adequately account for neuroplasticity and the recursive relationship between the brain, behavior, thinking, and feeling). This reality wasn't there to begin with, something investigators "discovered"; it is entirely man made, which we'll talk more about in chapter 5 on the social construction of reality.

Our journey will take us to the cutting edge of the fields of neuroscience, psychotherapy outcome studies, and postmodern theory and practice. It is from here that we will take the great leap into the language paradigm, the transformational domain of intersubjectivity, recognize psychotherapy as an art, and, finally, discover that coaching is a by far better metaphor for a empowering relationship. For the majority of the book I use the words "coaching" and "psychotherapy" interchangeably; both refer to the reflexive interplay of intersubjectivity and redescription. More on this later.

Though this book challenges the foundation of the mental health profession—the clinical/medical model—it takes what is good about the profession (many practical skills and perspectives) and simply, though profoundly, places them in a new context. This new context is that of human transformation or personal/spiritual growth. Yes, we are all in the same boat. And, of course, this puts an emphasis like never before on the personal or spiritual growth of the therapist.

Furthermore, "medical necessity" is as easy to establish and document as it was before; only now, being *bilingual*, we can just temporarily use a deficit language to describe the person we're helping (from a particular angle) for the purposes of getting insurance reimbursement. The same being true of establishing justification for government assistance.

At this juncture I need to explain an important caveat. Language is so powerful our care in its use is now paramount. I routinely place parentheses around "clinical" terms (e.g., "schizophrenia," "treatment," "medications"), or preface a clinical term with "so-called." This is to rob them of their reality and truth status. For the sake of readability I've had to leave out some of the parentheses and "so-called" prefaces. Also, the academic tone, especially in the beginning ("The Scientific Prelude") is largely to show how my conclusions follow from the latest neuroscience and psychotherapy outcome research. The rest of the book has a more personal and inspirational tone, apropos of what works in psychotherapy: connection (intimacy) and persuasion that engages both intellect and emotions.

I

The Scientific Prelude

ONE

The Structure of Social Scientific Revolutions

In his 1962 *The Structure of Scientific Revolutions* Thomas Kuhn introduced the idea of paradigm shifts in science that marked quantum leaps in knowledge interspersed among relatively long periods of what he called normal or puzzle-solving science. Normal science is where scientists work out the implications of the assumptions of the current and prevailing paradigm. During the process of normal science as technology and methods of analysis improve anomalies are observed to the point where they threaten the assumptions of the prevailing paradigm. For example, with the advent of particle accelerators we discovered that at very high speeds atomic and subatomic particles defy the laws of Newtonian mechanics. This breakthrough called for a new explanatory system, namely quantum mechanics. Examples of paradigm shifts are abundant throughout the history of science.

Though Kuhn used the word "paradigm" exclusively in reference to science it is commonly used in the social sciences. The word "paradigm" more generally means any coherent body of thought and associated practice that is based on certain assumptions. Or as Amy Blackstone (2012) puts it, a paradigm is "an analytic lens, a way of viewing the world and a framework from which to understand the human experience." The prevailing mental health paradigm that includes psychiatric diagnoses, neurofixity as represented by the "chemical imbalance" metaphor, and the representationalist view of language (i.e., that language represents rather than creates realities) falls under the social science paradigm of positivism. Blackstone outlines the commonly accepted social science paradigms as follows:

1. Positivism: the idea that there can be objective, value free, scientifically grounded knowledge
2. Social Constructionism: realities are socially constructed vis-à-vis cultural transmission
3. Critical: social and political forces shape a reality that is neither objective or value free; social justice being an objective of inquiry
4. Postmodern: there are no absolute truths; language creates reality

Social constructionism and critical paradigms are often included in the postmodern worldview, and we will do so here as well.

I think the use of the term "paradigm" is particularly instructive in describing the way in which one worldview gradually comes to subsume another worldview. In normal science there are relatively long periods of "puzzle solving." What are the brain markers for schizophrenia? What is the best treatment for PTSD? To what degree is bipolar disorder genetically determined? The list of "normal science" research is enormous, yet all the paradigmatic assumptions upon which that research is based are the same. Even the paradigm-incongruous exceptional research—be it complexity neuroscience, psychotherapy outcome studies, or postmodern theory and practice—is embedded in (or overshadowed by) the old paradigm in the sense that the old paradigm doesn't appreciate that this anomalous data is revealing signs of a completely new paradigm. Yes, even postmodern psychotherapy as it exists presently—far more theory than practice—is grounded in the modernist ontology (way of being). Nevertheless, it is the signpost of the new possibility, the vision of what will someday be a new embodied reality.

Paradigms by their nature cannot incorporate such anomalous information. Basic assumptions of paradigms are seen as absolute such that any contradictory evidence is seen for one reason or another as insignificant. In fact, more often than not, evidence that disputes a paradigm *cannot even be SEEN*. This is true because paradigms are made of words held together with certain assumptions and theories; said another way paradigms are vocabularies that cohere around basic theoretical assumptions and are self-affirming (i.e., everything is explained or rationalized within the paradigm). Thus in many cases we literally cannot see exceptions to the world revealed by the vocabulary, or if we do see exceptions they're only seen as insignificant (for one reason or another).

According to Kuhn, there is a tipping point when investigators are no longer able to ignore incongruous data and the fissures in the prevailing theory are too large, and simultaneously other competing explanatory systems begin to emerge.

This is currently the case with the mental health system. The new tide of paradigm-breaking research has come from the pragmatists (outcome researchers), postmodernists, and neuroscientists of the field. The pragmatic researchers who've been exploring the most relevant issue in psychotherapy, that is, its efficacy, have been gaining momentum in the past few decades. Postmodern theorists and practitioners have put the entire profession under historical, cultural, and linguistic scrutiny. And, finally, the neuroscientists have shaken the very foundations of the mental health profession with their discovery of neuroplasticity.

There is a wave of mounting evidence that is pointing in an entirely different direction; a new paradigm is emerging. Below is a summary of the past fifty years:

1. What works in psychotherapy is independent of the therapeutic model (Duncan et al., 2011).
2. Factors common to therapeutic efficacy all inhere in the subjectivity and dialogic skill of the therapist that include the ability (a) to form and maintain a therapeutic alliance, (b) to collaboratively yet persuasively articulate a more adaptive interpretation of the client's difficulty, and (c) to use real-time client feedback to alter the approach (ibid).
3. Psychiatric diagnoses have nothing to do with therapeutic efficacy (above) and, in fact, interfere with it (Bugental, 1987; Caplan, 1995; Grover, 2005; Duncan et al., 2011; Korteling, 2014).
4. The medical model is clearly *incompatible* with the emerging therapeutic ideals of strength-based, client self-determination, and wellness (Walker, 2006).
5. The DSM-5, the latest version of the DSM, has revealed the corrupting influence of the pharmaceutical industry on the formulation of psychiatric diagnoses (Frances, 2013a).
6. The self-fulfilling nature of psychiatric diagnoses is clear as daylight—for those who can see (Caplan, 1995).
7. The fact of neuroplasticity: the physical structure of the brain is reflexively related to thinking, feeling, behavior, and perspective. Causality goes in both directions (Begley, 2007; Schwartz and Begley, 2002; Siegel, 2012; Schore, 2012).
8. The discovery of neuroplasticity and the way the mind alters the brain is clearly in conflict with psychiatric diagnoses and the "chemical imbalance" theory that together comprise the centerpieces of the psychiatric model (Begley, 2007; Schore, 2012).
9. The field of epigenetics tells us that the expression of our genes (including those related to mental health) is highly influenced by our lifestyle, thinking, ability to solve life's problems, and emotional well-being (Lipton, 2008).
10. The domain of therapeutic change occurs in *intersubjective space,* which is facilitated by unconditional positive regard, accurate empathy, therapist authenticity (or congruence), attunement, right brain to right brain resonance, here-and-now presence, receptivity, and flexibility of responsiveness (Schore, 2012).

11. Postmodern literature reveals the power of language to create realities, identities, and power relations (Anderson, 1997).
12. Redescription or re-interpretation occurs *within the client's frame of reference* and is based on an egalitarian or subject-to-subject relationship. The language paradigm is crucial to the necessary interpretive flexibility (this book).

This is representative of the anomalous data that contradicts the prevailing clinical paradigm. These and other facts can no longer be denied, minimized, or ignored. The three areas of investigation and inquiry responsible for these facts are: neuroplasticity, pragmatism, and postmodernism. My own particular practical application of this new paradigm is what I call *postmodern coaching*. Taken together these form the basis of the transition of the mental health profession from an aspiring-to-be science to an art.

Moreover, we can no longer make "chimeras" out of the numerous new-old paradigm incompatibilities—either ignoring or not realizing the significance of the inconsistencies—which effectively hide what would otherwise seriously undermine the clinical worldview. This book will articulate a new paradigm that will incorporate and integrate these facts into a compelling new worldview. Putting the pieces of the puzzle together brings forth a coherent picture that reveals a whole new groundbreaking significance and profundity.

At this point it bears repeating that I'm not antipsychiatry. When it comes to psychiatric medications science and medicine give us basic (and important) guidelines based on human biochemistry and recommendations based on statistical studies. We need to take the Procrustean bed of medical "compliance" out of the psychiatrist's office. Furthermore, scientific research tells us what medication *might* work; relationship and communication tell us what *is* working—it's highly individualized. Psychiatry too is an art form.

I envision an artful psychiatry based on a collaborative relationship in which the client is a full partner (fully informed) in the experimental process of finding the best "medications" or discontinuing "medications." By its very nature a collaborative relationship has better communication; and isn't communication critical in the psychiatrist's decision-making? In an interview with Jeanie Lerche Davis (2007) for WebMD about "bipolar disorder," Carrie Bearden, PhD, a clinical neuropsychologist and assistant professor of psychiatry at UCLA, asserts:

> "We're really trying to understand what's going on *from the patient's perspective*. . . . The big focus is on developing a more individualized approach—not just prescribing a medication, but listening to the patient's feedback on various medications," she tells WebMD. "It's more of a team effort. *It's such an art,* not just finding the right medication,

> but finding the right dosage for that person, even using combinations of medications. (my italics added)

The space made for full communication is called intersubjectivity.

PARADIGM SHIFTS AND INCOMMENSURABILITY

The originality of this book lies in recognizing how the words and language we use, more than any other factor, powerfully determine the space of intersubjectivity, or the lack thereof. As will be discussed in the next chapter, the intersubjective field (aka intersubjectivity) is the space of intimate human-to-human contact where creative redescription and transformation take place; it is the "studio" of the *therapist-as-artist*. The main theme of this book is that the postmodern language paradigm is the lynchpin of intersubjectivity, and intersubjectivity is the key to neuroplasticity. The implication being that the selection and training of mental health professionals needs to be drastically altered.

As such, this book is an advancement in postmodern theory and practice in mental health; it is indeed a breakthrough in the postmodern approach. It is intended to reach the postmodern audience as well as those who are otherwise open-minded and committed to producing results in their work with people. This being the case, I need to address some concerns and considerations that could be leveled at what may look from the traditional paradigm to be a fairly polemical, unconventional, somewhat unacademic, and seemingly unempirical and biased work. The challenge becomes even greater when the paradigm shift is from science to art; yet as topsy-turvy and ironic as this may seem, the best neuroscience and psychotherapy outcome research validate this shift. In fact, the fact that psychotherapy is an interpersonal artform has been apparent all along (at least for those of a particular sensibility and discernment), only standing in the old paradigm we couldn't appreciate the full significance of this. Consequently, in order to facilitate the transition to the new paradigm I will need to devote part of this section to addressing the academic mindset.

This being an academic book the typical requirement is that this argument be balanced and situated in the existing body of knowledge in mental health. This is the standard and appropriate protocol of Kuhn's normal or puzzle-solving science. Normal science is situated within the existing body of knowledge; while being firmly rooted in it, it extends and elaborates on ("solves puzzles" in) the existing information in any given paradigm. Normal science research interprets and experiments within the same system of assumptions. However, as Kuhn pointed out, such puzzle-solving research often produces data that is inconsistent with the current prevailing organizing theory or paradigm. It is the anomalous data, the exceptions and contradictory evidence vis-à-vis the established body of knowledge, that leads us to the new paradigm.

This book is not about normal science as it would play out in the existing traditional body of knowledge in mental health. This book is about extending, interpreting, and drawing warranted conclusions about the current existing data that contradicts the prevailing clinical paradigm in mental health. In a sense, I'm "connecting the dots" that don't fit into the old paradigm; but as we will see, they form a striking new and profound pattern. Importantly, Kuhn maintained that old and new paradigms were fundamentally incommensurable in terms of methodology, worldview, semantics, etc. Kuhn (1962) relates:

> The normal-scientific tradition that emerges from a scientific revolution is not only incompatible but often actually incommensurable with that which has gone before. (102–03)

Incommensurable meaning impossible to measure or compare; lacking a common quality on which to make a comparison (*American Heritage Dictionary*, 2011).

As such, it's far more difficult to, in a spirit of impartiality, situate this material in the prevailing body of old paradigm literature. Moreover, when it comes to paradigm changes, there is no middle ground, compromise, or integration of paradigms; but instead, the old paradigm becomes a special case of the new paradigm. As we will see in subsequent chapters this attempt at integration—though it is perhaps an unavoidable step in the right direction—results in a modernist/postmodernist chimera (any mythical animal with parts taken from various animals, from *New Oxford English Dictionary*, 2001) that both conceals and stalls the growth of the postmodern language paradigm along with its power and possibility. In effect, the chimera is the old paradigm, in some logically inconsistent and superficial way, trying to *assimilate* the theory, perspectives, and practices of the new paradigm.

The current mental health paradigm (aka, medical model, or clinical paradigm, or "old" paradigm) can be summarized by the notions that psychiatric diagnoses are real, that assessment and diagnoses are important for "treatment," that the cause of psychiatric diagnoses is the chemical imbalance, that some people can't benefit from psychotherapy, that some people have "mental illness" and some don't, that theoretical framework is the most important variable in therapeutic outcomes, and that the human brain acts in a unidirectional and fixed way to affect behavior. Additionally, within the larger context of modernism of which it is embedded, the old paradigm views language only as representing "things" in the world (which we discover then label) versus creating realties (drawing and erasing distinctions with the use of language); in other words, language creates things as well as represents (names) them. Consequently, the old paradigm is a particular historically based worldview frozen in time—a perspective on the human condition mistaken for the whole. The postmodern language paradigm (or new paradigm) is free from such a rigid lens and, as we will see, frees the therapist to be fully in the present moment, receptive and responsive to all the subtle client-therapist emotional transactions, and free to maneuver in and out of the client's worldview in service of the intersubjective field so crucial for neuroplasticity.

As mentioned previously complexity neuroscience, psychotherapy outcome studies, and postmodern psychotherapies are the three areas of investigation that have called into question the very foundation of established thought in mental health. There are likely to be more than three, but these three pillars are sufficient to support the new paradigm presented in this book. These areas reveal the anomalous, exceptional, and contradictory empirical data that doesn't fit into the old traditional paradigm. In short, complexity neuroscience has resulted in the breakthrough of *neuroplasticity* in contrast to *neurofixity* (of which the chemical imbalance is an example). Outcome studies have demonstrated that the number one factor in the success of psychotherapy is the therapeutic relationship/alliance—the quality of which is a function of compassionate perspective, relationship skills, and skills in dialogue (in other words, nothing to do with diagnoses or theoretical orientation). Postmodern therapies have challenged the assumptions of the status quo from the outset and they've established a growing body of practice and interpretation that supports both neuroplasticity and the therapeutic relationship/alliance. Finally, all three converge in concluding that the intersubjective field is the crucible of human transformation wherein effective psychotherapy—as dialogic art form—takes place.

Thus we are making a paradigmatic leap out of the old framework, with its assumptions, presuppositions, and its logic of reductive theory, reductive empirical investigation, and reductive practice. As belief determines what we can see and can't see, comprehend and not comprehend, there's no way to fit this new paradigm into the old framework. In fact, the opposite is true: the old paradigm "fits into" the new paradigm.

Though different paradigms are incommensurable when treated as equals (in terms of comprehensiveness, explanatory power, and predictive power), they can be related when treated as unequals. In order to see how two different paradigms relate, let's take the analogy of the paradigm shift from Newton's mechanical model of the universe to Einstein's quantum/relativistic one. The quantum/relativistic model doesn't refute the mechanical model, it *subsumes* it, it incorporates it. The mechanical model involving such concepts as force, mass, acceleration, gravity, inertia, etc., holds true (for practical purposes) from a particular point of view. In other words, we run with Newtonian mechanics to build bridges, fly airplanes, etc. However, when we're looking at the very small (subatomic quanta) and very large (galaxies and bigger) the laws of mechanics don't hold anymore. The mechanical model is a special case of the quantum/relativistic model. Which perspective we take depends on the kind of problem we're trying to solve. We use quantum mechanics to create supercomputers and relativity theory to build global positioning systems. The "truth" is context dependent. Like quantum/relativistic theory did to physics the postmodern framework opens up the domain of human transformation into a new universe of principles and possibilities.

Likewise, postmodernism doesn't argue with the clinical world. From the postmodern perspective the clinical vocabulary in mental health is one point of view composed of words, concepts, beliefs, and practices (the integration of which is often referred to as a discourse). It is but one vocabulary among many vocabularies which attempt to address the dilemma of human suffering and transformation. No point of view or vocabulary is privileged nor absolutely right or wrong. The difficulty lies in that you have to be standing in the postmodern worldview in order to see this. The mental health profession in its current incarnation is a product of the modernist mindset and as such sees the clinical words, concepts, assumptions, and beliefs as absolute, essential, and objective realities. Herein abstractions are mistaken for entities. To say to the modernist clinician that "depression" is an abstraction and not a material entity is to say that the chair you're sitting on as you read this is not a material entity (which it indeed is). This is why the comprehension of this new postmodern framework (which is always a matter of degree) for the profession almost requires an ontological transformation of the individual (i.e., a shift in the way of being in the world). A person's subjectivity (her or his worldview), which is a function of his/her background experience, will or will not allow for receptivity to this point of view. Moreover, as we will later see with Michel Foucault, knowledge can't be separated from power—and the problem becomes even more intransigent. Importantly, our postmodern commitment to empirically established results forces us out of the yoke of doctrinal consistency, not into an "anything goes" framework, but instead into the search for a vocabulary (and practice) that is exquisitely receptive and responsive to its in-the-world effects—hence psychotherapy is an art form. The postmodernists/pragmatists use real-world practical results—both in terms of real-time psychotherapeutic practice feedback and in terms of outcome studies—as the criteria for the best working vocabulary (and corresponding practices). Onward to other potential criticisms emanating from the academic mindset.

The issue of *balanced* versus *biased* presentation is closely related to a change in paradigm. As is typical with Kuhn's normal science, foundational assumptions intact, theories vie for dominance and the best way to compete is to give opponent theories a fair hearing and then to address their weaknesses. However, having taken the leap into the postmodern language paradigm we're not arguing with the clinical interpretation; it's one of many ways of looking at people. The clinical world exists as a result of particular historically based assumptions, vocabularies, and practices. It is a point of view. We don't say points of view are wrong or right; but it only makes practical sense to evaluate them according to their consequences and utility. When it comes to paradigm changes the larger perspective/paradigm encompasses the smaller. Quantum/relativity physics doesn't argue with Newtonian mechanics, it includes it; it's just a bigger picture—likewise with postmodernism/neuroplasticity and the medical model in mental health. The only possible argument would be to insist that the clinical worldview was some absolute or essential truth/reality that we humans discovered (versus invented); in other words, the clinical worldview is not one among many interpretations. Later we will be discussing how history reveals the fallibility of our socially constructed truths (an activity sometimes referred to as historicism and deconstruction).

Another concern may be "Are philosophy and history relevant to clinical practice?" The answer is undeniably yes. As later chapters illustrate, philosophy and history allow us to see how human beings make things up as a function of historical contingency and utility, then forget that they made them up, then forever more view them as reality. As long as the clinical model is seen as objective reality (as a reality that exists prior to our languaging it, that we discovered and then described) then we will continue to be locked into the conceptual straightjacket that perpetuates normal routine science at the expense of a new paradigm of possibility. This is why the obvious harmful consequences of the medical model are not painfully obvious or are seen as unfortunate and unavoidable consequences of the clinical reality (e.g., the patient identity, chapter 9). This is why we haven't all prioritized "practice-based evidence" (versus evidence-based practice) the way Scott Miller and associates have. Normal science builds from and is contained within its presuppositional foundations. In order to free ourselves we have to see how and why these foundations were put together and how realities are socially constructed—this is the purview of history and philosophy. The resulting interpretive freedom gives rise to the flexibility and skill required to form and maintain intersubjectivity—the sine qua non of successful psychotherapy.

In this postmodern exposé have I ignored empiricism and logic? Absolutely not! In fact, the most important kind of empiricism is a foundational pillar of this work: psychotherapeutic outcome studies. In the pragmatist chapter (chapter 3) dealing with outcome studies I will propose that if the purpose of the mental health profession is to promote mental health (i.e., human transformation) then the priority of empirical research ought to be *outcome research*. This book distinguishes the essential perspectives, vocabularies, and practices that work in terms of making people's lives better. In fact, empiricism and inductive reasoning were meant to prioritize practical experience over pre-established categories, concepts, and beliefs; and the relevant practical experience is the therapeutic outcome (despite the difficulty in measuring it) and the observable practices and perspectives that produced that outcome.

A thesis throughout this book is that the clinical paradigm contains words and concepts that are seen as reality or truth (e.g., psychiatric diagnoses) and as such grounds our seeing and responding to our clients in terms of the clinical vocabulary. Consequently, the pragmatic, artful, experimental impulse to find and do what works—also at play in each individual psychotherapist's subjectivity—is forever constrained by this force that appears privileged as reality. This is significant because the best outcome studies to date conclude that therapist range and flexibility of receptiveness and responsiveness involved in a dynamic here-and-now dialogue are a crucial aspect of successful psychotherapy (Duncan, et al., 2011).

Freeing our helping relationships from hierarchical roles and liberating our therapeutic interventions from the dogma of the clinical vocabulary gives us a whole new world of wisdom and metaphor with which to flexibly experiment and interpret. This may be radical to say, but I believe the purpose of academic psychology/psychiatry is to produce more effective therapists and psychiatrists and not to maintain foundational paradigmatic consistency. In the postmodern world the only consistency we're looking for is finding the vocabulary and practices that allow us to repeat and expand on what works!

Does this work abandon science? No, in addition to outcome studies, it utilizes a new kind of science called complexity science and by extension complexity neuroscience. As far as reductionist and mechanistic science/neuroscience are concerned their application to a complex (versus mechanical) system, such as the human brain, is particularly problematic. As we will see in later chapters, properties that emerge with human language (itself an emergent property) feed back and allow the brain to put lower level (counterproductive) operations into perspective, thus creating the possibility for new action and corresponding neuronal networks. The mistaken application of reductionist science/neuroscience to human subjectivity and behavior is known as *scientism*. I will argue that complexity neuroscience—the human brain seen as a whole, as a complex system, in its social environment and with its adaptive capabilities—is the mental health profession's legitimate tie to scientific authority.

But what about evidence-based practices (EBPs)? EBPs are based on the assumption that it is the theoretical orientation and protocol (i.e., organization and techniques) that is the prime determining variable in the therapeutic outcome. Yet, the vast majority of therapeutic outcome studies show that therapeutic efficacy is independent of the specific theoretical approach (Duncan et al., 2011)! The therapist her/himself is the main variable and from a postmodern perspective this boils down to the therapist's subjectivity (i.e., worldview). The same is true for diagnostic-specific treatment protocols. Empirical outcome research has revealed that it is a false premise that we need to be wedded to theoretical orientation or consider psychiatric diagnosis when it comes to helping people. Ironically, the theoretical and diagnostic mindsets blind us to the relational, communicative, and non-verbal subtleties and nuances crucial in establishing and maintaining the intersubjective field.

It turns out there's another problem with diagnostic-specific treatment protocols. In reality a psychiatric diagnosis indicates a list of symptoms (impaired concentration, impulsive behavior, audio hallucinations, etc.). These symptoms—or better-said behaviors and subjective experiences—do exist, unlike the abstract labels that refer to them. So, in effect, the protocols are addressing the "symptoms"; but this one-size-fits-all mechanistic approach has many drawbacks. The main problem is that the diagnosis (and the role relationships inherent in the clinical model) blinds the therapist/psychiatrist to the far more important aspects of the client's subjective framework; for example, what the client's priorities are, their preferences, their concerns, their fears, their strengths, and, significantly, their responses to the therapist's/psychiatrist's emotive communications. Even a skilled and experienced therapist is always fighting the magnetic force of the clinical worldview of which the diagnostic-specific treatment protocol is embedded—so why not get rid of it?

In chapter 12 we will discuss how the therapeutic tools that already exist in the profession—including those within diagnostic-based or evidence-based strategies—can be employed far more effectively from within the client's subjective framework. Furthermore, as will be later revealed in chapter 3, the success of psychotherapy depends on two factors: the relationship/alliance (aka intersubjectivity) and the timeliness and fit of the reinterpretation of the client's experience. The critical skills and perspectives that support these factors are all but demolished by the inadequate and clumsy categories of "diagnosis" or "treatment protocols" (Bugental, 1987; Caplan, 1995; Grover, 2005; Korteling, 2014).

Finally, the one—albeit "meta"—way in which different paradigms *are* commensurable and comparable is in terms of real-world results. Vocabularies compete in terms of which better forward the quality of human life and humanity's civilizing discourse. Consequently, it is only empirical research in the form of outcome studies that will ultimately verify the practical truth of what I'm claiming about the postmodern language paradigm in this manuscript. Outcome studies have led us to the indispensability of intersubjectivity. But when it comes to the power of language, I admit that I have only my own personal and professional anecdotal evidence to point to. I will say that what has motivated me more than anything is the amazing results this framework has produced in my own professional practice (both public and private). Furthermore, witnessing the joy, the freedom, and the empowerment of clients freed from the clinical world has been a major inspiration in the writing of this book. Yet, the language paradigm has yet to be tested in terms of outcome studies. This book is a step toward such outcome studies. To quote Kuhn:

> However incomprehensible the new theory may be to the proponents of tradition, the exhibit of impressive concrete results will persuade at least a few of them that they must discover how such results are achieved. (1962, loc. 441)

This is my hope as well.

TWO

Neuroplasticity

Before I review the story of and scientific evidence for neuroplasticity I'd like to preface with three important points. Firstly, the notion that adult neuroplasticity has existed as long as human brains have existed. We don't need to be a neuroscientist to know that the *muscle memory* of an athlete or musician reflects new neural networks. Any adult that learns a new language or any other kind of skill is further evidence. With the right incentive and sufficient repetitive practice, though often difficult, people drop old habits and develop new ones all the time. Athletes and musicians through hard, repetitive practice permanently alter their performance. In her book *Train Your Mind, Change Your Brain* (2008), Sharon Begley illustrates how Buddhist monks through their mindfulness practice have shaped their brains in such a way as to be present to existence and largely experience expansive and positive perceptions and emotions. Somehow, in our reliance on science to tell us what is true we've lost sight of what's right in front of us. We don't need to understand the molecular characteristics that make clay pliable in order to make pots, statues, and cups out of clay.

With regard to neuroplasticity, what neuroscience really has told us is that the physical structure of the brain changes when we put in the attention and practice to alter our thinking and behavior. In other words, there are neurocorrelates to cognitive and behavioral change. Put the demand on the brain and it will change. The brain is an organ of adaptation; it even adapts to itself (e.g., in mindfulness training).

The second preface is that neuroplasticity is pretty much an established fact in neuroscience. In this chapter I have distilled the vast research on neuroplasticity down to the landmark studies that are often cited as key evidence for neuroplasticity. So for these two reasons—that adult neuroplasticity has always existed and is already a scientifically established fact—I'm going to emphasize how neuroplasticity has come to be the new metaphor in mental health.

Finally, I make the distinction between reductive neuroscience and complexity neuroscience. Reductive neuroscience (aka neuropsychiatry) is traditional neuroscience based on the view of the brain as a simple (versus complex) system, much like a machine with interacting parts. Like an automobile, the whole is simply the orchestration of all the interacting parts. When the machine is broken, fixing it amounts to replacing or adding parts. With the use of sophisticated instruments, reductive neuroscience looks to map the brain in great detail, right down to neurotransmitter levels. The tissue, neuronal patterns, neurotransmitter levels are then described with terminology that in effect fixes their description of the brain as if it were a static, unchanging organ—as if to "pin down" its structure and then compare "normal" with "abnormal" brains in order to see which parts need replacing. For example, when a neurotransmitter is at a lower than normal level, the reductive neuroscientists attempt to manipulate the brain in such a way to bring the level back up, i.e., put things back into "balance." Additionally reductive neuroscience claims that specific areas of the brain are locked into specific functions—lose the area, lose the function.

Complexity neuroscience, on the other hand, recognizes the brain as a complex system, as a functioning whole, including the brain's relationship to the body, other people, and its environment. Moreover, complexity neuroscience was born out of looking at the brain's ability to adapt to natural or artificial environmental demands as well as its ability to address itself using attention, mindfulness, redescription, and repetition (e.g., in the service of dealing with mental, emotional, and behavioral issues). Complexity neuroscience looks at the brain's adaptive potential. Neuroplasticity is a product of complexity neuroscience.

I will argue later in this book that in light of neuroplasticity, coaching (versus psychotherapy) may be a better metaphor for the helping relationship. Throughout the book I will sometimes use the phrase "complexity neuroscience" for a particular emphasis; however, for brevity's sake whenever I use the word "neuroscience" I mean complexity neuroscience.

EARLY INTUITIONS OF NEUROPLASTICITY

Before reductive and mechanistic science got its hands on the adult human brain, many researchers and thinkers speculated that the human brain was malleable. In 1793 while comparing the brains of trained and untrained animals, Michele Vicenzo Malacarne discovered that the cerebellum grows in response to training (Rosenzweig, 2007, 73). William James in his *Principles of Psychology* (1890, 104–27) speculated that the human brain is capable of reorganizing in response to repetitive operation (i.e., habit formation). Karl Lashley in 1923 discovered that the neuronal "movement maps" changed as an individual monkey's movement patterns changed; moreover the more frequent the movement, the greater the cortical terrain associated with that movement (Lashley, 1923, 585–602). In the mid-twentieth century, the Polish neuroscientist Jerzy Konorski (1948, 5) coined the term "neuroplasticity" in response to Donald Hebb's (1949) observation that repeated neuron-to-neuron transmission led to a kind of fusion of neurons.

THE BRAIN AS MACHINE

Santiago Ramon y Cajal's meticulous work in brain anatomy and function won him a Nobel Prize in 1906 as well as the title of father of neuroscience. In 1913 his *Degeneration and Regeneration of the Nervous System* (Cajal, 1913/1991) began a century-long hegemony of the static model of the adult human brain. Each anatomical portion of the brain had a specific sensory, motor, or intelligent function; ergo functionality lost by brain damage was functionality lost period.

Cajal's work launched a century of brain "mapmakers" analogous to the cartographic ocean voyagers of the fourteenth through eighteenth centuries. Notably were Paul Broca and his center for speech and Carl Wernicke's location of language. Soon an accomplished "map" of brain functionality emerged into the infamous "cortical homunculus" (a diagram) that shows the specific brain locations of sensory and motor functions. This was seen as the permanent anatomical arrangement of brain functionality. Some speculate that this arrangement mirrors the body parts' proximity in the developing fetus, thus fooling the cortical areas into thinking that adjacent fetal body parts in its contracted fetal position are contiguous body parts anatomically speaking and therefore map to adjacent cortical territory (Schwartz and Begley, 2002, 170). For example, in the contracted fetus the hands touch the face and correspondingly in the adult brain the sensory and motor areas of the hand and face are located next to each other.

Of course, the brain with fixed and immutable functional areas reflects the mechanistic and reductionistic worldview of the Enlightenment and subsequently modern medicine. The "chemical imbalance" metaphor was a natural extension of this brain-as-machine analogy—of course massaged, reinforced, reified (made into a reality), and made dogma by the psychiatric and pharmaceutical industries. This reductive neuroscience, alive and well even today, represents only part of the picture. To complete the picture we need complexity neuroscience with its interdisciplinary focus on the brain as a whole, in its relational context, and in its environment with demands placed on it including being challenged with mindfulness, new thinking, new language (redescription), and new behavior.

THE RELUCTANT PARADIGM SHIFT

Paradigm shifts occur by the gradual accrual of evidence that contradicts the prevailing paradigm, and neuroplasticity is no exception. Much of the research included in this section was dismissed or ignored by institutions and journals at the time of its release. It was only in retrospect that all the pieces of the puzzle came together to create neuroplasticity as a whole new paradigm of possibility.

Rather than give a detailed history, I'm going to describe four rough categories of neuroscience research that contributed to the establishment of neuroplasticity as a fact. We can think of these as the four legs that support the table of truth of neuroplasticity. These include (1) recovery of motor function (e.g., after a stroke); (2) sensory substitution: expansion of remaining sense mode (into the unused neural tissue) when another is lost (e.g., the enhanced hearing discrimination in blind people); (3) the neural correlates of habit; and (4) adult neurogenesis (i.e., stem cells in the brain producing more brain cells throughout the life span). All four involve the recruitment or creation of neuronal tissue to equip the body *to meet environmental demand*. For each category I will provide examples of research representative of that category.

For those interested in the story of neuroplasticity in detail I recommend *The Mind and the Brain* (Schwartz and Begley, 2002) and *Train Your Mind, Change Your Brain* (Begley, 2007).

Recovery of movement experiments typically use arms since both arms in humans and other primates are routinely used in normal daily activities. One arm's functioning can be lost due to stroke (in humans) or by experimental destruction of brain tissue called deafferentation (in primates). Recovery of motor functioning in the damaged arm is largely accomplished by restraining the functioning arm, thus leaving the subject to use the damaged (limp) arm to accomplish a task or a range of everyday activities. Usually a reward system is used to reinforce the agonizing incremental progress. Surrounding healthy cortical tissue reorganizes itself through the brain's integrative reach to the motor neurons of the affected arm in order to perform the function of the damaged brain tissue. The obvious example of this is the recovery of motion after a stroke (Bach-y-Rita, 1980; Taub et al. 1993, 347–54). Constraint-induced movement therapy is now a standard of care for stroke victims.

Sensory substitution happens when one sense (sight, hearing) is lost due to impairment of the sensory organ (eyes, ears) and the remaining sense organ through its sensory neuronal migration recruits the newly unemployed brain tissue (once used to operate the damaged sense organ before its demise) resulting in the enhancement of the remaining sense. Norihiro Sadato and colleagues (1996, 526–28) demonstrated that in blind adults the visual cortex (brain tissue normally used for processing visual images) had been re-employed to process both auditory and tactile information. This explains why even adults who lose their sight later in life have more refined peripheral auditory discrimination and heightened discernment and sensitivity in their braille-reading finger.

The fact that habits have neural correlates almost seems self-evident; however with the development of brain-stimulating movement maps and later of sophisticated brain imaging technology (positron emission tomography [PET], functional magnetic resonance imaging [fMRI]) it could be scientifically proven. Brown and Sherrington (1912, 250) and Lashley (1923) discovered that habitual movement was both cause and effect of neural networks. Later Konorski (1948), Hebb (1949), and Shatz (1992, 60–67) established the corollary notion that "neurons that fire together, wire together."

Finally, the discovery that the human brain generates new brain cells upon certain demands or opportunities, or just as a matter of course. Neurogenesis has been established in adult birds (Nottebohm, 1989, 74–79), rats and New World primates (Gould et al., 1997), and finally in adult humans (Eriksson et al., 1998). Fred Gage, member of the Eriksson team, speculated further that the adult human hippocampus might produce neural stem cells that would then migrate and integrate into existing neural circuits where they were needed. Eleanor McGuire et al. (2006, 1091–101) demonstrated this. She showed that London taxi drivers experience rear hippocampus enlargement; moreover, the greater the taxi driving experience, the greater the hippocampal enlargement.

Helen Neville, renowned neuroscience researcher, after accumulating almost a decade's worth of evidence that the auditory cortex can process visual input and vice versa (the visual cortex can process auditory information), concluded her address to the Dalai Lama:

> It is the outside world that determines the functional properties of the brain's neurons. And that's what our work has been about: how experience shapes the functional capacities of the brain. (Begley, 2007, 108)

Indeed, as Edward Taub famously put it, "It's all cortex" (Begley, 2007, 128).

NEUROPLASTICITY AND PSYCHOTHERAPY

The neuroplasticity mentioned above that heralded the new paradigm is referred to as "bottom-up" neuroplasticity. With bottom-up neuroplasticity the brain rewires in response to the organism's repetitive exposure to some outside demand or incentive (opportunity or punishment). From here on out we will be talking about "top-down" neuroplasticity. To put it simply, top-down neuroplasticity is where the mind and coordinated behavior change the brain. This of course leads us to the application of neuroplasticity, as the main operating metaphor, to psychotherapy. It is at this point where the practitioner supplants the researcher (with their PET and fMRI machines) and we enter the realm of psychotherapy as a dialogic art form where the medium is language and relationship.

The initial attempts at applying neuroplasticity to psychotherapy came in the form of mindfulness. Mindfulness is the primary transcendent practice in meditation or prayer, particularly in Zen meditation, which is exclusively mindfulness. Mindfulness is the practice of non-judgmentally observing your inner world of spontaneous feelings, bodily sensations, thoughts, and perceptions (often while focusing on a particular object or activity, e.g., breathing). It is sometimes called mindfulness-based CBT (cognitive behavioral therapy) when in addition to mindfulness skills we relabel or redescribe thoughts and feelings (such as "thoughts are not facts" or "that emotional overwhelm is a result of the lack of integration between the prefrontal cortex and the lower limbic system"). In actuality, we can dispense with the CBT portion as Buddhist practitioners routinely use analogies and metaphors to empower their observation of their inner world ("thoughts are like butterflies flying near us" or "our inner turbulence is like the stormy surface of the ocean").

Jeffrey Schwartz (2002, 71–88) at the University of California, Los Angeles (UCLA), reinterpreted obsessive-compulsive disorder (OCD) intrusive thoughts as "products of an overactive caudate nucleus" or "worry circuit" which can be observed on PET scans. Additionally, OCD thoughts were revalued as essentially "toxic waste from the brain." His therapy for OCD basically consists of practice using these new neuroscience-based interpretations to empower one's mindful detached awareness of obsessive thoughts and compulsive urges, then refocusing on more productive activities. For example, upon the triggering of a compulsion to avoid the cracks in sidewalks, s/he says, "This isn't an urge to avoid stepping on the cracks in the sidewalk; it's a faulty hyperactive brain circuit"; then s/he would practice mindful walking (in a detailed manner being aware of the sensation of walking while "batting away" spontaneous thoughts).

In 1996 Schwartz et al. (109) found that after ten weeks of his mindfulness-based CBT program twelve out of eighteen of his patients with OCD improved significantly. The improvements were matched by PET scans that showed equally significant shrinkages in the right caudate nucleus (the area of the brain that becomes enlarged with OCD). In other words, the physical structure of the brain changed measurably in response to changing the way people with OCD thought about their thoughts combined with the practice of substitute replacement behaviors. Subsequently, the UCLA OCD-clinic has treated hundreds of people a year (Schwartz and Begley, 2002, 91).

Teasdale et al. (2000, 615) trained their clients to view depressive thoughts as merely "events in the mind." They supplemented this interpretation with the assertions "thoughts are not facts" and "I am not my thoughts." By doing so they postulated that they could prevent normal sadness or frustration from developing into depression. After eight weeks of this mindfulness-based CBT program their 145 subjects (all having at least two episodes of major depression in the previous five years) showed a 45 percent reduction in the rate of relapse. This response was greater than psychiatric medications and any other form of psychotherapy. With the help of other confirming findings (Ma and Teasdale, 2004, 31), the conclusion was undeniable; mindfulness significantly prevents normal disheartening experiences from cascading into full-blown depression.

Mindfulness has since exploded onto the cultural scene in tandem with neuroplasticity. One of the reasons is that Buddhist monks have a near lifetime of practicing mindfulness and thus were natural subjects in the investigation of the relation of mindfulness and neuroplasticity. The Mind and Life Institute sponsors ongoing dialogue between Buddhist monks (including the Dalai Lama) and prominent neuroscientists (Begley, 2007, 11–15).

After the clear establishment of the fact that mindfulness and mindfulness-based CBT cause measurable changes in brain structure, other therapies, as if needing to prove their legitimacy too, have put their hat in the ring. In their chapter "Neuroscience: The Newest Force in Counseling and Psychotherapy," Allen E. Ivey, Michael J. D'Andrea, and Mary Bradford Ivey (2012, 49–52) review all the psychotherapies that have proven to reorganize the brain, including cognitive behavioral therapy, biofeedback, interpersonal psychotherapy, and EMDR (eye movement desensitization and reprogramming). They go further in pointing out that various therapeutic skills and intervention strategies have profound positive effects on neurotransmitter levels:

> There is a growing body of research literature on the neurobiology of psychotherapy that describes brain changes. These changes appear to be directly impacted by different psychotherapeutic processes . . . the types of changes clients hope to achieve in counseling and therapy are fostered by the neurological alterations that practitioners stimulate by using various theoretical principles, skills, and interventions that are increasingly known to stimulate the generation and optimal release of various neurotransmitters that promote changes in clients' neural wiring and brain functioning. (Ivey et al., 2011, 73, 52)

Another pioneering neuroscientist, Zindel Segal, puts it in reference to depression:

> Massive marketing has depicted the challenge in depression as one of correcting a chemical imbalance in the brain. . . . This may be true at the neural level, but we now know that there are multiple pathways to recovery, and a chemical imbalance itself can be restored in different ways. (Begley, 2007, 150)

Neuroscience has expanded the description of psychological problems beyond the "chemical imbalance" to include the entire brain anatomy. As we saw earlier with Schwartz's work on OCD, neuroscience-based therapies, not surprisingly, reinterpret psychological and interpersonal problems in terms of neuroanatomy. Daniel Siegel (2011) reinterprets an "emotional meltdown":

> The middle prefrontal cortex—the region that calms the emotionally reactive lower limbic and brainstem layers—stops being able to regulate all the energy being stirred up, and the coordination and balance of the brain is disrupted . . . we go down the "low road," moving directly from the limbic impulse to speech and action, and detouring away from the prefrontal "high road," where we are flexible and receptive rather than inflexible and reactive. We "flip our lids." (26)

Moreover, as we noted early from the Ivey et al. (2012) work, clinical researchers are recognizing many therapeutic techniques and strategies that alter neurotransmitter transmission and larger scale brain processes.

Note that as the *description* (or metaphor) changes so does the *prescription*. "Chemical imbalances" call for "medications." The integration of higher brain function (prefrontal cortex) with lower brain function (limbic system) in the pursuit of equanimity, empathy, and efficacy requires mindfulness and a host of other helpful therapeutic interventions. As Siegel (2011) relates:

> Many clinicians focus primarily on the concept of "chemical imbalance," and how various neurotransmitters, such as serotonin or noradrenaline, take you "up" or "down" as their levels rise or fall. However, I actually find that a deeper discussion of emotional regulation in the brain gives patients a larger view of the problem—and what we can do about it. (82)

Allan Schore (2012) adds to the chorus of complexity neuroscience researchers and practitioners that are challenging the prevailing paradigm that only pharmaceuticals can alter brain architecture and thereby produce the desired changes in emotional regulation and behavior:

> It is now becoming apparent that the idea that psychology (psychotherapy) changes the mind and biology (pharmacology) changes the brain and the body is outmoded. In 2005 the Nobel Prize–winning psychiatrist Eric Kandel argued there is no longer any doubt that psychotherapy can result in detectable changes in the brain (Etkin, Pettenger, Polan & Kandel, 2005). By 2008 Glass summarized the commonly accepted view: "Recent research in brain imaging, molecular biology, and

> neurogenetics has shown that psychotherapy changes brain function and structure. Such studies have shown that psychotherapy affects regional cerebral blood flow, neurotransmitter metabolism, gene expression, and persistent modifications in synaptic plasticity" (1589). In a 2010 neuroimaging study published in *Psychotherapy Research,* Tschacher, Schildt, and Sander asserted, "psychotherapy research is no longer concerned with efficacy but rather with *how effective change occurs*" (578). (10, Schore's italics)

Schore has been a major contributor to the toppling of the old paradigm and the building of the new paradigm. We all should now be concerned with "how effective change occurs."

We conclude this section with the scientifically backed assertion that psychotherapy produces significant and in some cases profound brain changes. This is true from the level of neurotransmitters to that of neural circuitry to that of the interaction of much larger brain components. Unlike the "shotgun approach" of powerful psychiatric medications (i.e., hasty, non-selective, indiscriminate, and haphazard; read: a partial cure with side effects), these brain changes are tailored to the specific subjective experience of the person as well as to their environmental challenges. Moreover because psychotherapy affects our *relationship* to our thoughts and feelings the results are often longer lasting.

ATTACHMENT THEORY AND INTERPERSONAL NEUROBIOLOGY

I want to preface the next section with the following caution against the ever-present temptation of reductionism (the use of oversimplifications and where a perspective on the whole is mistaken for the whole). Because of attachment therapy's focus on the reconciliation of early relationships, emotions, and the reenactment of formative patterns in the therapeutic relationship you might read the following passages and be tempted to say, "Oh, that's psychodynamic, object-relations therapy, or time-limited dynamic psychotherapy." Or, in response to attachment therapy's emphasis on non-judgmental empathetic receptivity and authenticity, you may want to say, "This is Rogerian." I caution against this because, like the blind men and the elephant, you'll mistake a perspective on the whole for the whole itself (the blind man touching the elephant's leg insists it's a tree). By labeling a part you lose the comprehension of the whole. This is very important in our consideration of psychotherapy as an art form whose medium is language and relationship.

The reductive mind is quick to proclaim, "There's nothing new under the sun." The postmodern mind sees it quite differently. The reductive and rigid nature of "theoretical orientations" prevents their fluid interplay and integration. If they're seen for what they really are, that is, vocabularies, then we're free to use the words, concepts, structures, and practices where and when they're called for, that is, artfully.

In the 1980s, Daniel Siegel, being disaffected over psychiatry's formulaic approach to mental health—DSM and medications—began to integrate neuroscience with attachment theory (Sykes Wylie and Turner, 2015). Furthermore, Mary Sykes Wylie and Lynn Turner (2015) point out that neuroscience and attachment theory were quite naturally coalescing disciplines and that consequently they mutually supported each other in their rise to popularity in the 1980s and 1990s:

> [I]t's . . . possible that attachment theory wouldn't have "caught on" if a virtual revolution in brain science hadn't happened at the same time. Bowlby always believed that attachment was biologically necessary in itself for survival. Looking at attachment through the lens of neuroscience from the late 1980s to the present, researchers found that the mother-child bond, in effect, began to knit together the neural filaments of the newly emerging baby-brain—literally altering both the structure and activity of neural connections. (4)

Siegel, along with other attachment theorists, believes that our first social bond (typically with our mother) served as the template for all subsequent relationships. It is in this primary relationship where we learn to regulate our emotions and empathize with others—to the extent that we do. And, of course, there are neural correlates to all of this.

As it turns out, all our subsequent intimate relationships amount to a struggle to repair that original bond; which includes, of course, psychotherapy. Sykes Wylie and Turner continue:

> Attachment research had emphasized the psychobiological core of attunement between mother and child—the continual, subtle, body-based, interactive exchange of looks, vocalizations, body language, eye contact, and speech. Attunement—or "contingent communication," as Daniel Siegel coined it—was really a highly complex, supremely delicate, interpersonal dance between two biological/psychological systems. If this contingent communication was a characteristic of healthy attachments between parent and child, or between husband and wife, or friend and friend, then wasn't it also critical to good therapy?

The new paradigm of psychotherapy as an art form means that we're now talking about very subtle and nuanced verbal and non-verbal interactions. The new therapist of the twenty-first century will have the sensitivity of a painter or sculptor, as opposed to the mechanical expertise of the automobile technician. To "become one" with another person requires interpretive freedom, a presence and receptivity, an ability to live in an indeterminate space where we can pivot on a dime, yet still respond in dialogue with our impressions. Whether we're talking about an infant or an adult with inflamed attachment bonds, the matrix of identity formation, emotional regulation, and greater personal authority is the same:

intersubjectivity generated and maintained by attuned, contingent communication. Siegel defines intersubjectivity as follows:

> Intersubjectivity: The shared experience created in the joining of two or more minds, revealing how the whole is greater than the sum of its parts. Intersubjective experience cannot be reduced to simply two subjectivities being added together; this is an example of interpersonal resonance. (2012, 467)

More on intersubjectivity later.

It should be becoming increasingly clear how the bulky, reductive, and totalizing labels and conceptualizations of the current mental health profession are indeed disabling in light of the sensitivity, flexibility, and responsiveness of intersubjective attunement. Through the clinical vocabulary we "see" broad categories: tangential speech, manic episodes, depression, unrealistic thinking, paranoia, tangential speech, manipulation, narcissism, histrionics, axis II, low self-esteem, co-dependence, cognitive distortions, a mentally ill person, "anxiety," emotional lability, etc. These labels by association bring other clinical categories of operation into play like assessment, diagnosis, psychiatric medication evaluation, case management, setting firm limits, consistency, etc. An observation of symptoms leads to assessment and diagnosis, diagnosis to treatment and the need for compliance. Interpretation and response are a unity, just different aspects of the same phenomenon. It's all very formulaic, you could program a computer to do it—and, believe it or not, some clever (but misguided) people are trying to institute computer therapy (Cartreine et al., 2010). Eliza[1] (Wallace and Dunlop, 2006) is even Rogerian! I hope you can see how the mindset and being of the artist and of the technician are worlds apart.

From the marriage of attachment theory and neuroscience—presided over by Daniel Siegel—came the birth of *interpersonal neurobiology*. The primary tenet of interpersonal neurobiology is that the personally and privately experienced mind is individually embodied and yet interpersonally constituted (i.e., created in relationship and communication)—a fact that took neuroscientists and a few discerning twentieth-century philosophers to discover. According to Siegel (2012, 6) the mind "is not separate from our bodies or from our relationships—it both arises from them and it regulates them." From our relationships springs forth our mind which then feeds back into our relationships. Additionally, and interestingly, Siegel has pointed out that the intrasubjective (within the mind) and intersubjective (between minds) attunement skills are the same and emanate from the coordination of the same neuronal structures and processes:

> Because it [the anterior cingulate cortex (ACC)] links body, emotion, attention, and social awareness, the ACC plays a key role in the resonance circuitry that lets us feel connected to others and to ourselves (In

> fact, the more we sense our own internal world, utilizing the ACC . . . the more we can feel the internal world of someone else). (Siegel, 2011, 125)

Psychotherapy, from the point of view of interpersonal neurobiology, reactivates our original attachment bond (usually with our mother) for the purposes of correcting earlier mistakes. According to Allan and Judith Schore (2012), the attachment, compassion-based felt relationship is the essence of the helping relationship:

> A central principle of our work thus dictates that attachment experiences shape the early organization of the right brain, the neurobiological core of the human unconscious (Schore, 2003). Indeed, therapeutic interventions are rooted in these same implicit dynamic relational processes. In treatment, these right brain affectively charged attachment experiences are communicated and regulated within the therapeutic alliance. The co-creation of an attachment relationship between the empathic social worker and the client has been seen as the sine qua non of clinical practice, and respect for the individual is, and always has been, paramount. (31)

According to Siegel (2012), the quality of attachment—whether mother/infant or therapist/client—is a function of attunement (or resonance). Attunement is the felt resonance of two subjectivities, a becoming one with another person. In Siegel's own words:

> Attunement is the way we focus on the flow of energy and information in an open and receptive manner. The circuitry of our own nervous system is such that if we attune, we come to create resonance in which our observing self takes on some of the features of that which we are observing. If we are attuned to another, this creates an interpersonal resonance in which each person feels felt by the other. (171)

Attunement is the gateway to intersubjectivity.

Siegel (2010, loc. 782) adds that attunement is dependent on the therapist's mindful presence, non-judgmentalness, and empathy. Attunement is (from the Sykes Wylie and Turner quote above) "a highly complex, supremely delicate, interpersonal dance between two biological/psychological systems." This "being with" rather than "doing to" (Bullard, 2015) is a completely new dimension in psychotherapy requiring vastly different skills, therapist worldviews (subjectivity), and education and training.

Intrapersonal attunement is recursively related to interpersonal attunement. This is part of interpersonal catalyzation of emotional regulation. When we communicate an authentically compassionate, connected, yet emotionally neutral response to the inner turmoil of another person, that person often then sees it in the same equanimous light. This is part of the unconscious resonance that we'll discuss later. In Siegel's words:

> Interpersonal integration stimulates internal integration. This is how interpersonal attunement catalyzes the interpersonal regulation [read: compassion, non-judgmental comprehension, empathy, respect for differences] that then becomes more autonomous self-regulation . . . interpersonal connections shape neural connections. . . . The brain influences mind and relationships; relationships influence brain and mind; the mind influences relationships and brain. (2012, 274–75)

Then the mindful therapist having sufficiently tuned into the client's world artfully brings his/her more pragmatic interpretive frame into the dialogic play in the form of redescription. And, as we will also see later, resonance (attunement) and redescription are mutually reinforcing. In fact, as is clear with Carl Rogers's work, empathetic responding can be a very subtle form of reinterpretation. Our efforts at trying to articulate our understanding of another's world is done with language and metaphor that can only approximate or even alter a client's meaning. Meanings and feelings are often ambiguous to begin with.

Siegel describes attunement as the empathetic, authentic, compassionate, and non-judgmental entering into another's world. Siegel's concept of resonance, i.e., "the coupling of two autonomous entities into a functional whole" (Siegel, 2010, loc. 1064), is a characteristic of *intersubjectivity*. In other words, we experience resonance in intersubjective space. The world of intersubjectivity is indeed dynamic.

But before we explore intersubjectivity further we have to get to feeling and subjectivity. Neuroscience, attachment theory, and psychodynamic theory came together to usher in what Allan Schore (2012) called an *affective paradigm*. Attachment and the new two-person psychology have everything to do with emotions and the unconscious. Breaking out of the cognitive paradigm (as epitomized by cognitive behavioral therapy) it looked like emotions were now *the* way. On the contrary, we'll see later that thinking and language are human culture's vehicles of emotion, passion, commitment, and transcendence. But whether we're talking about nature or culture, feeling or thought, unconscious or conscious what we're talking about is subjectivity. Subjectivity recognizes that thought and feeling are always linked. But first to feeling.

THE RETURN TO FEELING (AGAIN)

In Allan Schore's *The Science of the Art of Psychotherapy* (2012) he describes what he calls the *affective paradigm* shift within the mental health profession. Neurobiologically informed attachment theory tells us that an individual's identity integration and emotional regulation are a result of *interpersonal integration* based in very subtle, momentary, non-verbal, *felt*, and to a significant degree unconscious and recursive interactions. With the right relational stance and skill set, the mindful therapist—simply by being in relationship and in communication—results in a mindful client. Like the way tuning forks resonate so do human beings.

We're now entering into the intricacies of human bonds, relationships, and communications—which are profoundly *emotional*. Therapists must read and respond to (resonate with) very subtle emotional cues such as are expressed in the body and voice. Schore stresses that emotional resonance is a precondition for cognitive resonance. As a rough rule of thumb: right brain first (intersubjective attunement), left brain second (cognitive redescription). Moreover, much of the emotional resonance (or dissonance as the case may be) is happening on an unconscious level, often referred to as *unmediated* resonance (or dissonance).

For decades, in the midst of cognitive behavioral and managed care hegemony, the "black box" (to use Schore's term) of the unconscious was relegated to the sidelines of psychotherapy, much like the "black box" in commercial jets is not involved in routine daily operations. However, as we will see in our next chapter, outcome studies have for decades (by the way, the same decades) shown that the characteristically felt relationship and alliance are the overwhelming common factor in successful therapy, independent of theoretical framework. In response to this avalanche of evidence, the American Psychological Association has become increasingly interested in promoting education having to do with the role of feelings, therapeutic alliance, relationship, and therapist characteristics in the efficacy of psychotherapy. Schore relates his experience:

> In 2009 the American Psychological Association (APA) invited me to present a plenary address, "The Paradigm Shift: The Right Brain and the Relational Unconscious." In fact, that was the first time an APA plenary address was given by a member in private practice, and by a clinician who was also psychoanalytically informed. Essentially, what the APA wanted was something on the increasingly important role of affect in clinical and developmental psychology and neuroscience. (2012, 3)

This return to the unconscious or emotions marks the transition of the mental health profession away from its scientistic beginnings. *Scientism* is the misapplication of reductive science (and all its methods) to areas of inquiry where complexity science (or art) is called for. Human behavior and economics are two such areas, both of which, being products of the human brain (a complex system), are much better treated as art forms than sciences. Science and reason play a part, but only in the background, not the foreground.

As it turns out, this swing of the pendulum from reason to feeling happened during the nineteenth century in the romantic reaction to the Enlightenment. Between Immanuel Kant, David Hume, and the French Revolution (and later World War I) the universal hope that reason and science could be applied to the human condition and we would live happily ever after was dispelled. Kant's "Copernican revolution" demonstrated that the human brain cannot comprehend ultimate realities; thereby freeing space once again for metaphysics. Time, space, causality, and reason are evolutionarily derived categories of the human brain that are imposed or projected onto the physical world (Kant, 1772/1977, 35–43). Hume proclaimed rightly that "reason is the slave of passion." Finally, the bloodbath and irrationality of the French Revolution was in the name of the highest principles of human reason. When it came to the human condition, even human morality, we had to look to emotion. Passion and commitment were the feelings that compelled socially responsible (or enlightened) self-interest.

With the romantics, feeling, imagination, freedom from convention, passion, authenticity, morality, nature, individuality, and subjectivity took center stage. Commitment was the new authenticity. And, as we will see later, nineteenth-century Russian writers expanded and deepened the investigation of human subjectivity which eventually contributed to existentialism and further manifested in the psychological realism of the novel.

As we will see throughout this book the historical swing from objectivity to subjectivity is happening again. In the case of psychology, CBT—a preeminent objectivist/cognitive approach—is being challenged on many fronts. Even within the CBT movement preeminent practitioners have gone from investigating the realism of "hot thoughts" to changing our relationship to thought and feeling altogether in the form of mindfulness (Hayes, 2012). Acceptance and commitment therapy's (ACT; ibid) focus on value-driven committed action harkens back to the days of Goethe and Holderlin.

CBT is based in the medical model where the client is expected to fit into the structure of the CBT protocol and cognitions are "restructured" as if the process were a kind of mental surgery. As would be expected based on our discussion of alliance and attunement the structure and protocols of CBT wreak havoc on the relationship—except, of course, for those clients that are temperamentally disposed to adapting to roles; that is, they can play the expected role. Furthermore, CBT doesn't do anything to break the tie between feeling and circumstance, thus we are forever tied to examining thoughts/feelings by assessing how "realistically" they reflect our circumstances, thereby hopefully changing our feelings in the preferred direction. In contrast, the Eastern (in particular, Zen) perspective involving the radical acceptance of, selective indifference toward, and dissipation of feelings has been promulgated by thinkers such as Steven Hayes (2012; ACT), David K. Reynolds (1984; Constructive Living) and Eckhart Tolle (1997).

Psychodynamic or object-relations therapies are already situated to incorporate this new focus on emotion, attunement, and the unconscious. Allan Schore and Ruth Rosenbaum number among this group.

To summarize, the coalescence of attachment theory, complexity neuroscience, and neuroplasticity has brought emotions, the body, and the unconscious to the forefront. This most crucial domain in terms of therapeutic efficacy has been largely overlooked and thus undeveloped in the profession. Transference and countertransference are the two ancient categories that only touched on this. As it turns out if we add thought, perspective, and language into the mix we have all the ingredients of what we call subjectivity (that has emotional and cognitive as well as conscious and unconscious aspects). Eugene Gendlin (1996, loc. 442) in his focusing-oriented psychotherapy has long advocated that we not separate thinking from feeling from imagining from memory, nor divide conscious from unconscious—that they are in fact different aspects of a whole and unified experience. Moreover, it's clear to those sensitive to subjectivity that the connotative aspects of words are very much felt and, as such, are very much right brain and very much subjugating. Language (thought) versus feeling is a false dichotomy; ask any poet.

THE RETURN TO SUBJECTIVITY (AGAIN)

As mentioned above, subjectivity was part of the eighteenth-century romantic, nineteenth to twentieth-century literary, and twentieth-century existential movements. Subjectivity continues to the present day to be the central and seminal distinction in the postmodern worldview. In the twenty-first century objectivism turning in on itself—that is, science addressing the human brain free from the presuppositions of psychiatry—has culminated in interpersonal neurobiology which has, in turn, returned us to subjectivity. In other words, we were unable to escape the scientific-theoretical-objectivist-categorical frame of reference (like Swift's Laputins) until we turned it and its methods to the human brain. Through objectivity we rediscovered subjectivity. Kant did the same thing in philosophy.

More than a half a century after Carl Rogers (1961), the consummate artist of intersubjectivity, published *On Becoming a Person* neuroscience has returned us to subjectivity and intersubjectivity. As Allan Schore explained in a 2015 interview with Psychotherapy.net:

> Neuroscience has legitimized subjectivity in psychology and in therapy. Both science and clinical theory agree that psychotherapy is basically relational and emotional, and so we now think that emotionally and intersubjectively being with the patient is more important than rationally explaining the patient's behavior to himself. . . . In the critical moments of any session the patient must sense that we're empathically with them. Research shows a difference between the left brain understanding of cognitive empathy and right brain bodily-based emotional

> empathy. In other words, we're experiencing and sharing the patient's right brain emotional subjective states, being with the patient rather than doing to the patient. In this therapeutic context we have to also be in the right brain to make therapeutic contact, and for the patient to make contact with her deeper emotions. Later we may engage our left brains to more cognitively understand the emotional state. (Bullard, 2015)

Right brain first (intersubjective attunement), left brain second (redescription). Yet, aside from raw animal instinct emotion is always integrated with thought and language. This is the basis of culture or what Sigmund Freud called the sublimation of instinct. Subjectivity takes this into account; it implies an integration of feeling and thought. Interpretation or description is a coalescence of both cognition and feeling. Furthermore, when speaking of subjectivity we're also acknowledging that much of subjectivity is implicit or unconscious.

Moreover given the expansive, non-judgmental, empathetic, authentic, responsive, dynamic, unstable, and uncertain nature of the attunement process we are now in a place where the therapist's subjectivity is the crucial element in the healing process. Thus the logic is as follows. Therapist subjectivity—including mindsight (the ability to "see" the mind) or mindfulness skills—allows for attunement and attunement creates intersubjectivity, and it is intersubjectivity that is the transformative factor in psychotherapy. In Siegel's own words:

> When we use mindsight and its capacity to maintain an open stance to the internal world of ourselves and others, we are able to achieve attunement. . . . If we are attuned to another, this creates an interpersonal resonance in which each person feels felt by the other. The experience of joining two subjective inner worlds with each other is sometimes called intersubjectivity. (2012, 171)

Intersubjectivity, sometimes called the intersubjective field, is also the focus for some in the area of psychodynamic psychotherapy. Highly influenced by neuroscience, Ruth Rosenbaum (2012) has become one of our fellow travelers into intersubjective space. She emphasizes how *mirror neurons* are the biological basis of *unmediated resonance*:

> Our consciousness engages in Winnicott's "intermediate area" (1975) to such an extent that it is reasonable to postulate that all experience emerges from an intermediate, intersubjective space. What is this space like? A clue to the nature of intersubjective space can be found in the activity of mirror neurons, a type of premotor neuron first discovered in the mid-1990s in the prefrontal cortex in monkeys (Gallese, Fadiga, Fogassi, & Rizzolatti, 1996), and then in human brains as well. It was found that the same mirror neurons were activated not only when the monkeys executed certain actions but also when they observed the same action being performed by others. In humans, for example, if a person raises his hand, the same neurons fire in the brain of someone

> watching him as fire in the hand-raiser's brain. . . . They [mirror neurons] may be the neural basis for empathy, for our attainment to each other's inner states (Lacoboni, 2008). . . . According to Gallese (2003), one of the discoverers of mirror neurons, we all participate in a prereflective "shared intersubjective space" (160). The kind of empathy facilitated by mirror neurons suggests a possible "unmediated resonance" (Goldman & Sripada, 2005, 207) between human beings. (Rosenbaum, 2012)

Though it's clear that intersubjectivity has a boundary-less and involuntary aspect to it, I'm defining intersubjective space as a product of critical skills and perspectives, a co-creation that is highly dependent on the nature of the therapist's subjectivity. Intersubjective space is a *real experience,* we're clear when we're in it (and when we're not) and we're also clear as to the depth and breadth of it. So, in effect, we're taking a process that is already happening on a rudimentary level and maximizing its creative potential in the service of human transformation.

Siegel too has concluded that the therapist's subjectivity—by way of mindfulness and mindsight skills—is foundational in the therapist's ability to establish and maintain attunement with the client, as well as to resolve the inevitable conflicts that arise (formally called a corrective emotional experience). A corrective emotional experience—a term coined by Franz Alexander—is the surprise, relief, and insight we experience when another person doesn't confirm our default narrative-based negative expectations of him or her. As a therapist, facilitating a corrective emotional experience is important because misunderstandings and conflict require resolution if for no other reason than maintaining the quality of intersubjective space.

The therapist subjectivity required to acquire the critical skills needed create "attunement—or 'contingent communication,' . . . a highly complex, supremely delicate, interpersonal dance between two biological/psychological systems" (Sykes Wylie and Turner, 2015, 4) is hardly even on the radar in graduate selection and training of mental health professionals. James Bugental in his groundbreaking book *The Art of the Psychotherapist: How to Develop the Skills That Take Psychotherapy beyond Science* (1987) identified the rightful place of subjectivity in psychotherapy:

> We in Western culture are only now beginning to discover the primacy of our subjectivity. Yet life-changing psychotherapy is psychotherapy that engages the patient's subjectivity, and in that focus is its greatest difference from other psychotherapies. This focus calls for continual attention to the patient's inner experiencing, and it recognizes that the prime instrument needed for that attention is the therapist's own subjectivity. (3)

Bugental, not surprisingly, also recognize the need for a total transformation of selection and training of mental health professionals:

> We need to radically rethink the preparation of psychotherapists who will aid their clients in making major life changes. That work depends heavily on getting into the subjectivity of clients and thus calls extensively on the subjectivity of therapists. (1987, 268)

Rosenbaum summarizes the neuroscience call to new skills in the new domain of intersubjectivity (which the neuroscientifically informed, psychoanalytically oriented psychotherapists sometimes call the *implicit realm*):

> A question that needs to be further explored is what those personal attributes are and how people can learn to develop them. Siegel (2010) has elaborated on methods of cultivating aspects of the therapist's "presence" that contribute to attainment and resonance with the patient and has described the neurobiological basis for some of these aspects. Schore (June 2006), also speaking from a neurobiological perspective, cited the following traits as the most important in establishing the crucial right hemisphere to right hemisphere resonance between patient and analyst: the analyst's sensitivity, or "capacity to register respond to very slight differences or changes in emotion," the expression of affect, and a deep sense of devotion and commitment to the patient's well-being. . . . "All technique," he said, "sits atop the therapist's ability to access the implicit realm," the implicit realm of unconscious resonance and other forms of non-verbal communication. (13)

In other words, all therapeutic "technique" rests on, depends on, the therapist's "ability to access the implicit realm." Graduate training programs have "put the cart before the horse" in their emphasis on theoretical orientation and technique to the exclusion of the implicit realm of intersubjectivity and therapist subjectivity. In some graduate programs therapist subjectivity is addressed in a very general way in terms of the therapist's own personal development, self-reflection, insight, self-awareness, self-actualization, etc. The nuances and subtleties of attunement or creating intersubjective space—"therapist's presence . . . capacity to register respond to very slight differences or changes in emotion"(from Rosenbaum quote above)—are new critical dialogic skills and are not even known in graduate training, except in very rudimentary training in listening and empathetic responding. Judith and Allan Schore (2012) and James Bugental (1987) describe the sensitivity of the psychotherapist as artist:

> In previous writings A. Schore (2003) describes the operations of the therapist's right brain by which the sensitive clinician's oscillating attentiveness is focused on barely perceptible cues that signal a change in state and on non-verbal behaviors and shifts in affects. In discussing "the art of psychotherapy," Bugental (1987) stresses the importance of the sensitive clinician's ability to "learn to experience finer and finer distinctions or nuances." He states, "The primary instrument brought to the support of the client's therapeutic efforts is the therapist's

> trained, practiced, and disciplined sensitivity. In many ways, this sensitivity is akin to a musical instrument which must be carefully prepared, maintained, tuned, and protected" (222). The clinician's capacity for intersubjective communication depends upon her "being open to intuitive sensing of what is happening in the back of the patient's words and, often, back of his conscious awareness" (Bugental, 1987, 11). (Schore 2012, 43)

Anyone familiar with the mindset and skills manufactured out of most graduate programs in psychology, psychiatry, or social work can now see that therapists are indeed educated and trained—through the emphasis on theory, technique, diagnosing, etc.—to be veritable "bulls in china shops." Evidence-based practices suffer from the same problem.

Also what's completely new—addressed in this book—is how the clinical vocabulary is constitutive of the therapist subjectivity (or worldview). Allan Schore's (2012) book is aptly named, *The Science of the Art of Psychotherapy*. Though he's *pointing at* the art, he's still standing on and observing from the clinical (pseudo-scientific) worldview. Let's take the following quote:

> A. Schore describes the nature of the implicit and explicit processes in the psychotherapeutic context:
>
> During the treatment, the empathic therapist is consciously, explicitly attending to the patient's verbalizations in order to objectively diagnose and rationalize the patient's dysregulating symptomatology. But she is also listening and interacting at another level, an experience-near subjectively level, one that implicitly processes moment-to-moment socioemotional information at levels beneath awareness (Schore, 2003, 52). (36–37)

As we will see in subsequent chapters, the use of words and concepts like "objectively diagnose," "patient," "treatment," "symptomatology" clearly indicates the clinical worldview that always takes center stage, thus precluding the delicate unpacking of the person's subjectivity. The therapist's expert stance (i.e., diagnosing) delineates a domain of relevance that relegates the emotional realm of the person's subjectivity to the background, thus leaving it unattended, or, at best, under-attended. What's really happening in this hypothetical scenario above is that the therapist is picking up on the implicit level the client's reaction to being positioned as "patient" which always skews the unfolding of his/her subjectivity. This passage exemplifies the "chimera" (spoken of earlier) composed of incompatible paradigms, the problematics of which cannot be fully appreciated absent sufficient grounding in the postmodern language paradigm. The course of the conversation would be very different if the clinical agenda was absent and the client co-determined the direction of the conversation and domain of relevance as is integral to a subject-to-subject, human-to-human, egalitarian relationship. The delicate and responsive dance between client and therapist that privileges the client's self-determination is aptly described by Carl Rogers after a demonstration interview in 1986:

> Whatever else is evident in this interaction is that the client knows best. . . . You don't consciously know where you're going, but if I can just trust that and just be with you on each strange step of the way, why it will lead somewhere. Just to be a little absurd. If I had had some goal for this interview, it would have completely wrecked it. (Natiello, 1996, 127)

Facilitating the unfolding of another's subjectivity is a process involving great skill, timing, initiative, restraint, spontaneity, artistry, sensitivity, emotional expressiveness, reflection, awareness, and verbal acuity. This process is far more like musical improvisation, where spontaneous communication of emotions and instrumental technique is integrated with spontaneous responding to other musicians—an intimacy that's hard to describe and exhilarating to experience.

On the other hand, the "chimera" demonstrated in the Schore quote above illustrates how a well-intentioned therapist can think s/he can have a "foot in both worlds," when in fact s/he does so only at the expense of the efficiency and efficacy of the entire process. The content of what the interpersonal neurobiologists are saying is right, but they can't see the self-defeating context (the scientific-medical vocabulary, the academic tone) in which they're saying it. These revolutionaries are pointing in the right direction but they have their feet firmly planted in the "rock hard" apparent realities of the clinical world.

The language of most academic and scientific literature is characteristically dry, often soporific. This type of writing presupposes that reason and argument are the means toward truth and truth will set us free. This is true in the domain of objectivity, not subjectivity. Reason and the scientific method have their uses, for sure. But the pre-Socratic view that poetry—an artful use of language and metaphor—has an important truth of its own, especially in the domain of human subjectivity, is the point we're trying to revive.

As long as the clinical worldview is seen as an objective reality it cannot be addressed and deconstructed out of the therapist subjectivity and therefore stands as an insurmountable obstacle to the intricate subject-to-subject communication needed for attunement, resonance, and the attainment of intersubjective space, the final frontier.

THE BLACK BOX

The standard form of neuroplasticity research is to repeatedly challenge the brain with adaptation (e.g., the loss of sight), repetitive movement, or some mindfulness-based behavior change and then observe changes in

PET or fMRI scans. In other words, produce the desired change in behavior then check to see how the brain reorganized to accomplish it. The point I'm trying to make is that the accomplishment of the behavior change is good enough! The brain may as well be a kind of mysterious "black box." Our job from here on out is to by trial and error create the conditions—in terms of perspective and practice—that produce the desired changes. This book through its condensation of complexity neuroscience, psychotherapy outcome studies, and postmodern theory and practice has identified these critical conditions as intersubjectivity and redescription.

Complexity neuroscience has brought us the malleability of both brain and subjectivity which is a breakthrough paradigm that has revealed a new frontier in mental health. But that is as far as it goes. From here on out to advance the profession we're looking for perspectives and modalities that resonate with the brain as a complex and malleable organ. We now know that language, thought, and mindfulness are the new medium of the art form of psychotherapy. Transformative communication is a function of relationship, appropriateness, timing, poignancy of metaphor, languaging, passion, and perspective. I call my work postmodern coaching to emphasize this.

The practitioner's relationship with complexity neuroscience brings to mind the Zen parable: "Don't mistake the finger pointing toward the moon for the moon." Neuroscience has pointed us to the reality of neuroplasticity, subjective plasticity, and the possibilities for human transformation that they bring. We need not keep examining "the finger doing the pointing." Neuroplasticity is a fact; the question now is what practices and perspectives create the intersubjective space and problem redescription necessary to facilitate subjective and practical empowerment in the people we meet with.

So we conclude this section on neuroplasticity with the primacy of the development of the therapist's subjectivity as the means of empathetic, non-judgmental presence, authenticity, receptivity, and contingent communication—approaching a kind of oneness with the client while maintaining distance sufficient to engage the emotions in reinterpreting the client's experience. This is a very dynamic form of therapy that requires moment-by-moment receptivity and responsiveness both intrasubjectively (within the mind of the therapist) and intersubjectively (between therapist and client). Therapist subjectivity and therapeutic intersubjectivity are recursively related.

In chapter 11 ("A Postmodern Narrative—the Subjectivity of Compassion") we will introduce a multidisciplinary worldview that serves as an example of how a big picture supports being a big person in service of the embodiment of authentic non-judgmentalness, unconditional positive regard, and a wide-angle empathy so crucial in a therapist's subjectivity.

These qualities are not something that can be willed out of nothing, nor do they occur naturally with little or no effort (e.g., wisdom that comes with age), nor are they taught in graduate school, nor can they be pretended, nor are they the result of some privileged access to absolute or metaphysical realities. They are a result of a deliberate and prolonged multidisciplinary investigation into the human condition.

As it turns out the pragmatists, led by Scott Miller, have also discovered that the research bears out that the therapist's subjectivity is the key variable in the success of therapy.

NOTE

1. The computer therapist accessible on the web, see Wallace ad Dunlop (2006) for web address.

THREE

The Pragmatists

The pragmatists are those researchers and practitioners willing to use hard data to see if psychotherapy works, and if so, what about psychotherapy makes it work. This started with early outcome studies (e.g., Landis, 1938; Denker, 1946; Wolff and Precker, 1952; Eysenck, 1952; Rogers and Dymond, 1954). In the 1980s this project improved with meta-analyses, among which Smith and Glass (1977, 752) were prominent. Since then extensive reviews and analyses have been published (e.g., Lambert et al., 2004; Wampold, 2001). The results were positive for psychotherapy, but in particular for the *common factor* (what was common among all therapeutic orientations) of the *therapeutic relationship* (Grencavage and Norcross, 1990). In their introduction to *The Heart and Soul of Change* (2nd ed.; 2011), Barry Duncan, Scott Miller, Bruce Wampold, and Mark Hubble summarize the psychotherapy outcome research of the last several decades:

> Of those factors directly related to treatment outcome, one of the largest contributors to outcome is the therapeutic relationship, which encompasses a wide range of variables found among therapies, no matter the therapist's theoretical persuasion. Therapist-provided variables, *especially the core conditions popularized by Rogers (1957),* have not only been empirically supported but are also remarkably consistent in client reports of successful therapy (Norcross and Lambert, 2005). (loc. 1239, my italics added)

I've italicized the reference to Carl Rogers's core conditions—unconditional positive regard, accurate empathy, and therapist congruence (or authenticity)—as part of my emphasis throughout this book of the critical importance of his work. References to Rogers's core conditions are replete throughout the literature of psychotherapy and they are especially central to the three pillars—interpersonal neurobiology, outcome studies, and postmodern therapies—supporting the new social constructivist (aka linguistic) paradigm. In the chapter on the subjectivity of compassion I maintain that the presence and coalescence of Rogers's core conditions in the being of the therapist is a function of a multidisciplinary perspective on the human condition; a way of being acquired through years of transformative work, not something that can be intuitively grasped and then acted out. Again, we're talking about the therapist's ground of being: subjectivity. We extend Rogers's work by adding the authentic, timely, and artful integration of human wisdom in to the client's subjectivity. All this in service of the therapeutic relationship.

Norcross (2011) borrowing from Gelso and Carter (1994) uses the following definition of therapeutic relationship:

> We can operationally define the client-therapist relationship as the feelings and attitudes that therapist and client have toward one another and how these are expressed. (296)

Take note at how close the relationship defined as "feelings and attitudes" above is to the attachment theory emphasis on the felt relationship (right brain to right brain resonance) between participants. The felt quality of the bond, as well as the maintenance of this bond through occasional corrective emotional experiences, is the foundation. How a therapist "feels" toward a client is not addressed in graduate training programs, except by way of addressing "countertransference" as a means toward getting a handle on negative feelings toward the client—hardly sufficient.

Integral to the therapeutic relationship—and to some degree synonymous with it—is the therapeutic alliance. The therapist-client relationship is a purposeful one based on a mutual commitment—a commitment to the quality of human life in general, and a commitment to the quality of the client's life in particular. In addition to professional, ethical, and legal parameters, this is the framework that holds the relationship. Therapeutic goals that derive out of this commitment vary from the very subjective (identity integration, feeling better, emotional regulation, etc.) to the very practical (better relationships, professional advancement, obtaining the practical necessities of life, etc.) or both. Not surprisingly the quality and strength of the therapeutic alliance is highly correlated with therapeutic success. Duncan et al. (2011) continue:

> Evidence regarding the power of alliance is reflected in more than 1,000 findings (Orlinsky, Ronnestad, and Willutzki, 2004). Researchers repeatedly have found that a positive alliance—that is, a partnership between the client and therapist to achieve the client's goals (Bordin, 1979)—is one of the best predictors of outcome (Norcross, 2011; Horvath and Symonds, 1991; Martin, Garske, and Davis, 2000). (loc. 1224)

Importantly whether we're talking about the therapeutic relationship or therapeutic alliance (note: throughout the rest of this book we will be using relationship and alliance synonymously and interchangeably) the critical determinant is the quality, especially in terms of feeling, of the therapeutic dialogue.

Scott D. Miller, PhD, and his colleagues have worked tirelessly over the past several decades to ferret out from research, experience, and feedback what works in psychotherapy. They discovered that successful psychotherapy was indeed independent of therapy modality and instead dependent on the relational skills (sometimes referred to as "common factors") of the therapist. These skills include the ability (1) to form and maintain a therapeutic alliance; (2) to facilitate client participation and engagement; and (3) to be able to persuasively convey a more adaptive interpretation of the client's challenge (Duncan et al., 2011, 1507–2351). Furthermore, Miller et al. (2013, 89) elaborate further that these relational skills involve very subtle and reciprocal transactions between therapist and client—that therapy "is a fluid, dynamic process, one involving a complex and nuanced series of interchanges" and as such, therapy needs to be correctly understood as a craft.

It is here that we have a startling new connection. The therapeutic alliance is an intimate collaboration between therapist and client which is highly dependent on (1) the relational stance of unconditional positive regard, accurate and felt empathy, and therapist congruence/authenticity, and (2) the dialogic skill of moment-by-moment presence, receptivity, and responsiveness of the therapist. In other words, the conditions of the therapeutic alliance (Miller's, Lambert's, and the American Psychological Association's emphasis) are the same as those for the creation of intersubjective space (Schore's, Siegel's, and Rosenbaum's emphasis). So the new connection I'm making is between the therapeutic alliance and intersubjectivity. They're different aspects of the same thing. In general, the therapeutic alliance (more about doing) emphasizes practical problem solving. Intersubjectivity (more about being) emphasizes identity integration, relational bonds, and emotional regulation. The therapeutic relationship, therapeutic alliance, and now intersubjectivity are the universally agreed upon essential ingredients of successful psychotherapy.

Client engagement, another important distinction mentioned above, is implied in the dynamic, empathetic, fluid, collaborative, receptive, and responsive nature of the therapeutic dialogue as well as the therapeutic alliance. Relationship, alliance, and engagement all imply client participation. Intersubjectivity implies dialogue and dialogue implies client participation. The creation of intersubjectivity is the creation of space for the client's voice, or said another way, the unfolding of the client's subjectivity. The vulnerability in our relational stance (mentioned above) creates the room for the client to be vulnerable, and similarly with authenticity. The creation of intersubjective space (and therefore the therapeutic alliance) is a very intimate, dynamic, dialogic, recursive, felt, and non-verbal process. This is the nature of right brain to right brain attunement.

In both interpersonal neurobiology and psychotherapeutic outcome research therapist characteristics, sensitivity, attitudes, relational skills, dialogic skills, and perspectives are increasingly being seen as the basis upon which the alliance/relationship and therefore success of therapy depends. According to the 2006 APA Presidential Task Force on Evidence-Based Practice:

> Central to clinical expertise is interpersonal skill, which is manifested in forming a therapeutic relationship, encoding and decoding verbal and non-verbal responses, creating realistic but positive expectations, and responding empathetically to the patient's explicit and implicit experiences and concerns. . . . Research suggests that sensitivity and flexibility in the administration of therapeutic interventions produces better outcomes than rigid application of . . . principles. (2006, 277–78)

It then follows that the formation and maintenance of a therapeutic alliance (intersubjectivity)—being a function of dialogic/interpersonal skill—is highly dependent on the therapist's frame of reference. We recall the postmodern insight that perspective and action (including speaking and listening) are always in accord with each other; thus the therapist's worldview and moment-by-moment "showing up" will determine her/his actions and his/her interpersonal skill. The APA Presidential Task Force continues:

> Because of the importance of therapeutic alliance to outcome, an understanding of the personal attributes and interventions of therapists that strengthen the alliance is essential for maximizing the quality of patient care. (2006, 278)

In other words, the fluidity, dynamism, flexibility, presence, responsiveness, along with the compassionate, empathetic, and authentic (what we might call Rogerian) framework emanate (or not) from the therapist's subjectivity ("personal attributes" or "personality" being a reflection of subjectivity). Intersubjectivity is dependent on the character of the therapist's subjectivity. The therapist's subjectivity must be constituted (i.e., made or created) such that it can reach and resonate with the client's subjectivity. This is what I call working within the client's frame of reference.

Furthermore, whether we're talking about integrating the functioning of the brain, resolving our attachment bond issues for the sake of emotional regulation or relationship harmony, or solving practical problems the necessary and sufficient conditions are the same: intersubjectivity constituted by context (unconditional positive regard, accurate and felt empathy, and therapist congruence/authenticity) and content (the very dynamic, dialogic, and nuanced therapeutic dance).

In addition to all the felt, compassionate, empathetic, and authentic qualities of the therapeutic relationship necessary for attunement and resonance emphasized so far, Wampold (2011) points out how important it is for the therapeutic alliance that the therapist provide problem redescriptions which also resonate with (if not emerge from) the client (the third of Miller's common factors or relational skills). In other words, the timing, flexibility, and range of the therapist's interpretive capacity are crucial. Bugental (1987) writes:

> Whatever the theoretical perspective of a depth psychotherapist, she must continually maintain some awareness of the patient's inner flow of experience. The most exquisitely crafted interventions are futile and often counterproductive—when advanced with timing and form that fit poorly with where the patient is in his subjectivity. (10)

As might be considered obvious, empathetic attunement (intersubjectivity) is a precondition for interpretive resonance *and* interpretive resonance strengthens empathetic attunement. Said another way, when a therapist offers a new interpretation of a client's situation that fits well with the client's frame then the client feels additionally acknowledged, validated, heard, or just plain gotten!

Putting it all together. We have the crucial three elements of therapeutic success on (1) the relational stance of unconditional positive regard, accurate and felt empathy, and therapist congruence/authenticity; (2) the dialogic skill of moment-by-moment presence, receptivity, and responsiveness of the therapist; and (3) interpretive flexibility and range needed to facilitate interpretive resonance or fit. Of course, these three elements overlap and are recursively related, but I think this division best supports translating this into practice.

Often I will abbreviate this trifecta as (1) intersubjectivity and (2) interpretive resonance. In intersubjective space the client is perfect as she or he is. We're not trying to go anywhere, we're just being with. This is the Rogerian non-directive stance that involves the three Rogerian conditions and the dialogic skill (1 and 2 above). When we add redescription (3 above) we enter more the realm of doing and thus are more in the domain of therapeutic alliance.

Implicit here is the fact that the one-size-fits all vocabulary of the Diagnostic and Statistical Manual (DSM) or of any given therapeutic modality (psychodynamic, cognitive behavioral, etc.) is a Procrustean bed[1] upon which the client must fit even if need be forcibly "stretched," which is a Pyrrhic victory at best, moreover, practically guaranteed to sacrifice the alliance (except in those cases where the therapeutic modality resonates with the worldview of the client). In other words, absent a therapeutic alliance and the intersubjective field what we have is the Nietzschean clash of wills where one participant must prevail and the other must either submit (euphemistically called "compliance") or rebel (aka non-compliance).

Yes, believe it or not this is what is going on, on the often unconscious or subconscious feeling level, beneath the "polite," "professional," "rational," and "explicit" surface of psychotherapy and psychiatry as they're currently being practiced. From the postmodern point of view "compliance" is winning the battle at the cost of the war. Yes, this is the source of all the complaining, commiserating, and labeling that therapists and psychiatrists do. The vast majority of therapists and psychiatrists have never been trained on how to work collaboratively within the client's frame of reference and to privilege client choice. Embodying the Rogerian core conditions involves a lifetime of personal transformation and professional training.

As we will mention again in later chapters once liberated from the rigid categories, formulations, and protocols of the clinical worldview, the therapist will be free to artfully experiment with empowering vocabularies and practices in order to find those that *fit the client*. The reason being the clinical worldview or theoretical ontology (Heidegger, 1927/1962) doesn't allow us to learn from our experience. Again like Swift's Laputins we can't see what's painfully obvious right in front of our noses because we see through the self-affirming categories and presuppositions of the clinical worldview. Coarse (clinical) distinctions dominate at the expense of fine distinctions. Clues as to what works and doesn't work are subtle, and for the artist it is these "clues" that we experiment with in order to ultimately flush out what works in each uniquely individual relationship. For example, don't most wise or prudent people (e.g., experienced and accomplished teachers or sports coaches) already know from experience what *we* need outcome studies to tell us, i.e., the importance of the relationship and alliance (though they may not use the term "alliance"). Outcome studies tell us what is already obvious.

The other breakthrough Miller and his group have made is to recognize psychotherapy as a *craft* (or art form) whose development involves (1) establishing a baseline of the therapist's competence (according to the criteria above), (2) implementing systematic and frequent feedback, and (3) using deliberate practice as a means of incorporating feedback into a new skill (Miller et al., 2013). In the introduction to *The Heart and Soul of Change*:

> Unlike a manufacturing operation, with linear inputs and predicable outputs, therapy is a reciprocal process, in which the inputs are changed in and by the participants' interaction. . . . The eventual form a treatment assumes is thus entirely dependent on the materials available; the skills of the artisan; and most important, the desires and preferences of the end user. (Duncan et al., 2011, loc. 1166)

Isn't this another way of saying "contingent communication: a highly complex, supremely delicate, interpersonal dance between two biological/psychological systems" to use Daniel Siegel's term? As we'll recall from our discussion on interpersonal neurobiology, attunement is a highly reciprocal or recursive process.

Whether we're talking about emotional regulation, harmony in relationships, corrective emotional experiences (attunement and Siegel), or solving practical problems (alliance and Miller), the relationship and therapeutic skills are strikingly similar. Furthermore, both approaches conclude that the being or subjectivity of the therapist is the most crucial factor, because it is the subjectivity of the therapist (constitutive of both professional and personal worldviews) that either supports or precludes the creation of intersubjectivity—attunement and alliance—with our clients. Judith and Allan Schore (2012) assert the primacy of the therapist's subjectivity in the right brain to right brain attachment process in the development of a therapeutic alliance:

> Scaer (2005) describes essential implicit communications embedded within the therapist-client relationship:
>
> Many features of social interaction are non-verbal, consisting of subtle variations of facial expression that set the tone for the content of the interaction. Body postures and movement patterns of the therapist . . . also may reflect emotions such as disapproval, support, humor, and fear. Tone and volume of voice, patterns and speed of verbal communication, and eye contact also contain elements of subliminal communication and contribute to the unconscious establishment of a safe, healing environment (167–68). (Schore 2012, 36–37)

These right brain communications convey expressions of "the personality of the therapist" more so than do conscious verbalizations

Implicit communication is happening on a felt level often, if not always, below our threshold of awareness. You can try to hide your personal and clinical judgments, but the unconscious knows better. The body imposes its communications on "the other" regardless of our conscious intention. The subjective framework of the therapist is often filled with relationship-toxic personal prejudices, embodied normative social judgments, and professional-clinical stereotyping labels.

Amazingly despite the competency of the professional *role* it is the subterranean, partly conscious, partly unconscious, right brain to right brain felt relational resonance that is determining the outcome of therapy! As it is practiced currently, empathy and unconditional positive regard conveyed in therapy are almost always partial or inauthentic expressions.

In other words, the therapist's authenticity when it comes to unconditional positive regard and empathy is crucial. In chapter 11, "A Postmodern Narrative—the Subjectivity of Compassion," I will offer a multidisciplinary historically based narrative/perspective that is meant to support this ever so elusive alignment of the Rogerian conditions.

Yet, a therapist can't "see" her/his subjectivity. What they perceive (both as obviously or tentatively true), what they attend to, don't attend to, think, feel, say (including the words they use) or don't say, and do (including bodily and otherwise non-verbal communications) or don't do are a direct result of their subjectivity. Subjectivity resembles captivity. Because client characteristics are the basis of psychiatric labels (statistically formulated), client characteristics (appearing as "symptoms") trigger by association the psychiatric labels, psychological interpretations, and the entire clinical worldview. Once this happens the therapist/psychiatrist thinks they're "observing" the client from a neutral standpoint. This is an exacerbation—due to psychology's fallacious tie to scientific objectivity—of the normal human tendency to think we're seeing people, unmediated, as they are.

Recall from the Schore quote above that on the explicit level the therapist is "objectively diagnosing." What the professional "sees" is "flat affect" indicating psychosis, "poor hygiene" indicating depression, "manipulation," "entitlement," "paranoid ideations," "manic behavior," "delusional thinking," "unrealistic thinking," "cognitive distortions," "hyperverbalness," "anxiety," "grandiosity" indicating "bipolar mania," someone who hasn't been "taking their medications," a person with a "mental illness." The actions that correspond to this clinical languaging are formulaic, template, one-size fits all: psychiatric medication management, cognitive behavioral therapy, "life skills," and various strategies to alleviate "symptoms." Actions are in perfect accord with the way things show up. Interpretation and response are a unity, just different aspects of the same phenomenon.

In other words, at the level of subjectivity the person trapped in the clinical worldview is just as delusional as a person filled with imaginative and unfounded systems of belief. Both are immune to modification based on evidence or efficacy. The only difference is that of consensus. There's more than a little irony here. Can sixty million Frenchmen be wrong? Consensual delusions abound, ask any advertising executive, ask Edward Bernays (the father of public relations and the nephew of Sigmund Freud)—the government and corporate world profit handsomely from this fact.

While all this "treatment" is happening, the professional is completely oblivious to the verbal and non-verbal expressions and clues indicating the client's subjectivity, preferences, concerns, priorities, ambivalences, fears, desires, commitments, and subtle responses to her/him. Because "therapy" is something "done to" the client the client's *responses* to the therapist's statements, questions, and interventions go practically unnoticed. What the professional is concerned with is compliance, not resonance.

From this seeming "neutral" vantage point the therapist has hidden thoughts and feelings (sometimes below the threshold of awareness) about the client. The therapist's *being* is now split. On the one hand, there is the professional role presented and on the other hand there is the private clinical assessment and other judgments going on in their head.

Many of these private thoughts in the form of judgments and complaints are often shared with friends, spouses, colleagues, and in supervision—this is when the therapist is being authentic or congruent.

This bifurcation of the therapist into role and feeling is what Carl Rogers referred to as therapist incongruence or what we postmodernists call inauthenticity. What essentially happens is that the modern alienating world has been replicated in the therapy session—complete with inauthenticity, the need to "look good," manipulation, antagonism, and the power struggle to define or be defined, submit or dominate. Mechanical empathy doesn't help. Alliance, connection, intimacy, unconditional positive regard, collaboration, authenticity, felt and accurate empathy—and consequently attunement, resonance, contingent communication, and intersubjectivity—are all precluded by the medical model and the clinical ontology (way of being).

Thinking that you're objectively observing or "assessing" a client (the basis of "doing to" a client, aka intervention or treatment) has profound consequences. Blind to the subtleties and nuances of recursive right brain to right brain felt transactions, a therapist is oblivious to the ways in which his or her felt experience (and corresponding actions), the setting, the protocol, and role expectations all create what he or she is "observing"—not the least of which is the self-fulfilling nature of psychiatric diagnoses and clinical vocabulary in general, as we will discuss in chapter 5 ("The Social Construction of Reality") and chapter 9 ("The Creation of the Patient"). The fact is people are different and experience themselves and their world differently in different settings and with different people. Quantum mechanics applies here: the observer effects what's being "observed." A colleague of mine and I used to marvel at how different our "clients" looked at the shopping mall adjacent to our clinic; when they arrived in our waiting room they mysteriously transformed into "patients"—the setting called for that role. Not recognizing this phenomenon and not leveraging it has devastating consequences for the therapeutic relationship and its outcome.

Like my caveat regarding the firmly established fact of neuroplasticity, the same is true of what works in psychotherapy. The evidence is overwhelming that the nature of the therapeutic relationship and therapeutic alliance are by far the most crucial factors in psychotherapy success. For a more thorough exposition of the research supporting this I recommend *The Heart and Soul of Change* (2nd ed.; 2011) by Barry Duncan, Scott Miller, Bruce Wampold, and Mark Hubble. The purpose of *this* book is to translate this into *practice* and to look at how language and paradigm profoundly impact these essential factors.

It should be becoming increasingly clear that to get to what works in psychotherapy through the maintenance and enhancement of intersubjective space and the therapeutic alliance is a completely new paradigm involving vastly different skills. You can't have a foot in both the clinical world and in the world of the client because the clinical world is categorical knowingness (diagnoses, symptoms, as well as the huge assortment of clinical terminology and interpretations) as opposed to the unknown universe of our client's unique world. Furthermore, this kind of expansive inquiry is going to take an alert mindfulness in order to avoid our "knowing" (in the form of both thought and perception) with any kind of certainty our client's experience. Feeling a bit unmoored. Good, that means you're getting it!

Yes, the twenty-first-century psychotherapist (or coach) will be more like Stradivarius in making violins than a manualized car mechanic. In art and craft we become one with another person; the mechanic assessed the "object," diagnoses, and treatments. Training will be a much more intimate process. The psychotherapist will be trained in heightened sensitivity and making subtle intrapersonal and interpersonal distinctions. Now we're talking about feedback-informed practice in real time, just like any other art form. You're welcome APA.

What's missing from both the interpersonal neurobiologist and pragmatists is the very foundation of the brain's subjectivity and capacity for change: language. Moreover, both of these camps at best retard, at worst bollix up their efforts with the clinical and scientific vocabulary. It would take the postmodernists to finally address the power of language.

NOTE

1. A structure or schematic to enforce strict application of a method based on the Greek myth of Procrustes, who stretched or chopped off the limbs of travelers so that they could fit on his bed.

FOUR

The Postmodernists

One might justifiably question why the postmodernists are included in the scientific prelude, as postmodernism has clearly undermined science as a source of absolute truth. The reason is that in my twenty-five years of interfacing with postmodern psychotherapists I've never met one—with the possible notable exception of Michael White—who has escaped the gravitational pull of the clinical and/or academic world and traversed into the linguistic paradigm (part II). The result is a kind of weird chimera composed of postmodern notions resting on a modernist ontology (or way of being). Postmodern therapies as they currently exist represent a transitional stage toward the linguistic paradigm.

The postmodern philosophical movement began with Friedrich Nietzsche's (1901/1968) *perspectivism*—the idea that there are no absolutes, no "thing in itself," no metaphysical world; but instead all there is is perspective. Putting it simply, Nietzsche asserted, "There are no facts, only interpretations." Martin Heidegger (1959/1971) and; Ludwig Wittgenstein (1922) added the primacy of language: "We don't use language, language uses us" and "The limits of my language means the limits of my world," respectively. Søren Kierkegaard (1846/1992) proclaimed, "Subjectivity is truth." Michel Foucault (1983) emphasized how knowledge and language are instruments of power.

For our purposes I'd like to use Jill Freedman and Gene Combs (1996) definition of postmodernism or the postmodern worldview: (1) Realities are socially constructed; (2) realities are constructed through language; (3) realities are organized and maintained through narrative; and (4) there are no essential (absolute) truths. Adding further, we *experience* a reality yet we don't experience the linguistic architecture that created the reality in the first place. A world appears and we are simply subject to that world. Our perceptions, feelings, thoughts, and behaviors are perfectly in accord with the world that simply "shows up." Interpretation and response are a unity, just different aspects of the same phenomenon. We speak a world into existence to which we are then subject—only to have forgotten our authorship! One can surmise why the postmodern worldview is so difficult to grasp.

Around the 1980s postmodern ideas began to influence psychotherapy. With their focus on language, postmodern therapies attempted to defy the prevailing realities (psychiatric diagnoses and therapist with expert truths with which to define the client) of the mental health profession. Solution-focused therapy focused on exceptions to the problem or on a desired future. Narrative therapy externalized the problem, decentered dominant cultural discourses, and empowered clients' preferred narratives. Collaborative language systems recognized that each of us instantiate systems of language and the trick is collaboration. The common theme is the privileging of the subject's/client's worldview as well as the claims that reality is a construction of language and the language of the dominant cultural discourse supports and reflects power imbalances in society.

The postmodern practitioners were by default pragmatists (in the philosophical sense of the word as well). Postmodernism is like a very unstable intermediate compound in a chain of chemical reactions—it's a point of view that, practically speaking, can't stand on its own for very long. The privileging of all points of view as valid quickly leads to moral relativism and nihilism. Utility or *what works* becomes the obvious criteria for choosing among perspectives or vocabularies. The questions of utility for whom, social context, and grand narratives are for another day and perhaps another author. But as far as the mental health profession is concerned utility is self-evidently defined in terms of which perspective, vocabulary, and practices are going to facilitate our helping people feel better, achieve their goals, or, in general, improve the quality of their lives as they envision them. What's new from a postmodern light (at least ideally) is that we no longer see the psychologistic vocabulary (e.g., Diagnostic and Statistical Manual/ International Statistical Classification of Diseases and all its ancillary words, concepts, and practices—see chapter 6) as objective reality or absolute truth—it's just one among other competing vocabularies. The clinical vocabulary's (medical model's) pseudo-link with science does not exempt it from being a cultural artifact, i.e., being one vocabulary among others. We're no longer fixated, like some private investigator, on discovering some essential truth (diagnosis, unconscious dynamics, hidden motivations, resistances, defense mechanisms, "how they really feel," etc.) of which the client him/herself might not even be aware. John Walter and Jane Peller (2000), prominent innovators in solution-focused therapy, put it like this:

> From our reading of postmodern philosophy and pragmatism, we decided to abandon the debates over epistemology and the debates over the foundation of knowledge. Taking his cue from Nietzsche and William James, the contemporary author of the new pragmatism, Richard Rorty, suggested: "Instead of saying that the discovery of vocabularies could bring hidden secrets to light, [the pragmatists] said that new ways of speaking could help us get what we want" (1982, 150). So, instead of asking, "How do we know what is real about the client?" we have decided the more relevant question is "What do our clients want and what new ways of speaking or conversing might help?" (32)

So clearly the postmodern perspective adds a very unique element to both interpersonal neurobiology and the pragmatists. Though both emphasize the dynamic, egalitarian, empathetic, authentic, non-judgmental, felt-relationship, collaborative, and dialogical connection between therapist and client, neither explores the primary impediment to this. The postmodernists broke through into the language paradigm. Language is the medium of both thought and interpretation. Language defines our possibilities and our limits. When the interpersonal neurobiologist redescribes (reinterprets) "Obsessive Compulsive Disorder" as a "faulty cingulate gyrus" it creates an identity separate from the compulsion as well as an opening for committed action that wasn't there before. The pragmatically minded therapist can't be restrained by the "theories" and "orientations" (languages or vocabularies) of psychotherapy when looking to align and collaborate with the client's frame of reference. Even our ability to open-mindedly get feedback from our clients—in the form of a questionnaire or real-time nuanced non-verbal feedback—is highly dependent on being relatively-speaking free of prejudices, presuppositions, and professional vocabularies.

I could have easily added the works of Carl Rogers and Thomas Szasz as two other domains in psychology converging on and contributing to this new paradigm. Rogers was quintessentially postmodern in his person-centered work, in particular the three conditions for successful therapy he espoused: accurate empathy, unconditional positive regard, and therapist congruence (authenticity). Szasz was definitively postmodern in his understanding of language and power. So it is here that I leave these two titans of humanism. Both men had the vision of postmodern freedom, but neither had sufficient vocabulary to articulate a coherent and comprehensive framework sufficient to fundamentally break with the old paradigm. I'm eternally grateful to each.

THE RESONANCE BETWEEN POSTMODERN THERAPIES AND COMPLEXITY NEUROSCIENCE

Anyone who has practiced any of the postmodern therapies (solution-focused therapy, narrative therapy, or collaborative language systems) has doubtless experienced many miraculous changes in their clients. Yes, focus and languaging are that powerful.

As it turns out, I believe part of their success has to do with the way these approaches more realistically address the brain as a complex system, as an organ of adaptation, and as capable of self-regulation. Moreover, they take advantage of neuroplasticity by virtue of their focus on incremental change.

All postmodern therapies privilege the client's point of view, preferences, desires, goals, concerns, temperament, interests, and passions. So right off the bat, in an Aikido like way (see chapter 13, section "Aikido—The Way of Unifying with Life Energy"), we're working within the brain's well-worn neuronal patterns.

In solution-focused therapy we find exceptions to the problem (i.e., times when the problem is less severe or less frequent) and find out what thoughts, attitudes, words, behaviors, and circumstances resulted in that relatively positive outcome. In other words, we find out what our client is already doing that works! Just by us focusing on what's working our clients begin doing the same in some kind of virtuous cycle! Often our sessions become a recounting of what worked during the week followed by an analysis of why things went well. The traditional solution-focused homework is to continue to notice what's working better and do more of that. Solution-focused therapy's focus on incremental change nicely matches the way the brain forms new neuronal networks incrementally through repetitive practice. The approach is highly individualized, including working closely within the client's neuronally based motivational structure.

Narrative therapy takes advantage of the brain's ability to have multiple identities and narratives that support those identities. It also challenges our received interpretive frameworks when they're not serving us or our relationships. Yet, what most amazingly mirrors the brain as a complex system is the narrative therapy technique of *externalization*.

We've already discussed Daniel Siegel's mindsight skills. Without attention to our inner world of subjectivity we are dominated by the momentary contents of our inner world (thoughts, feelings, images), mainly because we identify with those contents and see them as true or reality. As it turns out another postmodern revelation is that we can choose what to identify with and oppose that which we choose not to identify with. For example, we can identify with our commitment and oppose the negativity (negative thoughts and feelings) that would otherwise sabotage our commitments.

In narrative therapy we externalize the thoughts/feelings that support undesirable behaviors or habits. We externalize the problem. People aren't the problem, the problem is the problem. What this does in neuroscientific terms is pit the higher order brain functioning against the lower order brain functioning. By naming (externalizing) the inner subjective experience of the lower brain function the person can identify when it is starting to take over. Having and externalizing conversation about the effects of "the problem" furthers this separation and makes "the problem" easier to identify and transcend. Here's an example.

I once worked with an eleven-year-old boy who had an anger problem. Apparently the problem was so bad that for years prior the county awarded "wraparound services" in order to help him and his mother. I was very touched when in our second session he, while crying, said, "I don't want to be a mental patient all my life." Yet, it seemed to his mother that he hated her and the rest of his family. It was clear that the little boy was both the "identified patient" and the "identified problem." Both the boy and his family despaired at his inability to "control his anger" (bad languaging). The problem was that when the anger was triggered the child identified with the anger and its justification. Externalizing to the rescue.

During the second session we began to talk about the anger as if it were separate from him. When does the anger take you over? What does it force you to do? What triggers an invasion? How does it trick you into cooperating with it? I playfully grabbed a pillow and pretended it was anger trying to take him over, he beat it with his fists with enthusiasm! For the first time in his life he had an ally against the anger; it was him and me against the anger!

At the third session both the boy and mother reported things were much better both at home and school. We talked of the numerous times he resisted the anger and kept it from taking over him. When I asked him, "How did you do it?" he said, "I realized my anger was the enemy not my family!" We spent the rest of the session talking about what he was going to be when he grows up. There were a few tune-up sessions after that. We had accomplished in five sessions what a psychiatrist and an army of social workers weren't able to do in several years! By clearly identifying the limbic (emotional) process as it was immediately experienced we were able to engage the neocortical (higher reflective) process in labeling it, contextualizing it, and transcending it.

Collaborative language systems, as the name implies, recognizes that our subjectivity is intersubjectively constituted (i.e., made or created). In other words, everything we privately subjectively experience—including our perceptions, thoughts, feelings, beliefs, values, etc.—is a product of our communications with others. Human beings are language systems whose origins span both space and time. We will recall that this is a pivotal recognition in complexity neuroscience. Interpersonal neurobiology is based on the understanding that the human mind is a product of relationship. Indeed, the brain, mind, and relationship are all recursively related—they all mutually influence one another. Daniel Siegel calls the brain, mind, and relationship a triangular unity where information and energy flow between them:

> [O]ne reality with three facets—not three distinct domains of separate realities. . . . We see the emergent process of mind as being embedded in the triangle. We cannot separate these three elements of energy and information flow from each other: They are three facets of one reality. This is not a dualism (or trioism); rather, this is a "monism" in that we see the one reality as being energy and information flow patterns. The three primes of experience—the irreducible aspects of the system—are mind, brain, and relationships. There's no need to find a way to simplify this triangle, to reduce one element into the other. (2012, 26–27)

One of the things that clearly astounded me a couple of decades ago when I started practicing postmodern therapies was how unnecessary the entire clinical vocabulary was. It was clear to me that with the right focus and language you could get the job done better and faster. But, more than that, the clinical worldview with its focus on and language of disorders, illness, and deficits was clearly creating a problem that didn't exist prior. Our clients, as all human beings, clearly had problems. But the way the problem or situation was languaged, defined, described was clearly up for grabs. In my individual and group sessions we simply stopped using the language of pathology and started using the language of empowerment. Then all the miracles began to happen. Unexpectedly, though, I found myself a stranger in a strange but wonderful land. There was no question that, though I still showed up at the clinic, performed my sessions, did my paperwork, signed-in and signed out, made small talked, and attended meetings, I was undeniably inhabiting a new reality.

All three postmodern therapies came out of philosophically informed experimental efforts that were honing in on practical results. As it turns out, when you focus on strengths, exceptions, solutions, unique outcomes, preferred life narratives, heretofore transparent influence of dominant cultural discourses, client interests and passions you get better and quicker results. As I mentioned before, I believe this to be true because they resonate with the human brain as a complex system.

The days of institutional benign neglect so necessary for this kind of experimental process, so necessary for results-based learning may be gone as the vice of institutionalized evidence-based practices tightens.

THE CLIENT AS EXPERT: A HISTORICAL TRANSITION

Carl Rogers, the majority of postmodern therapists, and much of the coaching profession are firmly entrenched in the client-as-expert paradigm. Postmodernism as a whole is allergic to any privileged or universal narrative (or truth), thus giving rise to the primacy of the individual's subjectivity. From this standpoint the therapist's expertise lies in bringing out the client's expertise in getting in touch with and learning to interpret their own experience as well as creating their preferred lifestyle and reality (frequently involving resisting the forces of conformity). This is essential for persons to enter the experimental and artistic frame of living. The point was to liberate the individual from normative or prevailing cultural discourses, to have a voice, to think for him or herself.

I believe this to be a historical transitional step, largely in reaction to the insidious and pervasive way in which social discourse—largely directed by those in power—constitutes our minds. Our seemingly private thoughts, feelings, and values are not so private. Discourse is the phenomenon of language, meaning, and practice as they coalesce and are transmitted between persons—much like memes (defined as the basic units of culture), only broader and more encompassing. Needless to say, the client as expert standpoint is something we must forever be vigilant to protect as dominating discourses are transparent and live in the very words and phrases we speak!

Traditional psychology, psychiatry, and social work were (and still are) unwitting agents of these subjugating normative discourses. And, as we have seen, they added their own special touch—the *pathologizing vocabulary*. Any psychological theory (vocabulary), as we will see in the next chapter, is also imposed (literally just in the speaking, it's very insidious) on the client at the expense of the client's interpretive independence. The client-as-expert stance was clearly a crucial advancement and is still a very legitimate approach.

The client-as-expert stance is clearly an aspect of intersubjectivity. It's implied in the relational stance we refer to as subject-to-subject or human-to-human. We need to be well practiced and possess some degree of mastery in being able to suspend our frame of reference in order to enter a not-knowing position; this is the basis of accurate empathy and true curiosity. On the other hand, we do know, things do occur to us from within our frame of reference and depending on the degree of our own transformation and embodiment of human wisdom, we may have a lot of pretty important things to say. This is where persuasion, deliberate influence, and inspiration come into play. And because such insights at least in part derive from and are integrated with the client's frame of reference they are essentially reinterpretations or redescriptions. Of course, not all our experimental redescriptions are suitable to our clients and this requires interpretive flexibility, privileging the client's responses, and a commitment to the integrity of the intersubjective field. Said another way (with some poetic license), our reinterpretive work is always within the client's frame of reference. Intersubjectivity is the basis of and foundation for redescription. The client determines the suitability of means and ends. We have to stay relevant to the client and not vice versa. The distinction and mastery of intersubjective space—of course with the help of others—is the built-in safeguard to avoid as much as possible the therapist's colonizing tendency. This is quite a journey as our cultural agency is transparent to us.

This is a very tricky area as in the beginning a therapist is all too ready to bring on untimely and ill-suited advice, opinion, intervention, strategy, etc. The honing to and maintaining of intersubjectivity is a very refined sensibility. This is why the therapist's subjectivity is of crucial importance and therapist selection and training should reflect this priority.

The groundwork has been laid, now it is time to talk about the elephant in the room. Though these three cutting-edge areas of investigation are all pointing to it—and here I would include Steven Hayes and acceptance and commitment therapy—they can't recognize that what's missing and what's being called for is the language paradigm. In my experience even most postmodern practitioners haven't yet taken this final leap out of the psychologistic vocabulary and/or its scientistic/academic framework. Either once again the forces of conformity and convention are in play, keeping a foot firmly and comfortably in the clinical vocabulary, or there is just something plain mysterious about human subjectivity that allows for the coexistence of two clearly incompatible paradigms, or both. It's as if the Newtonians agreed with the conclusions of quantum and relativistic theory but still went on to force the entire universe into the framework of Newtonian mechanics while somehow in their subjectivity were able to ignore or minimize the anomalous data.

This is important—and this is why I'm writing this book—because the great power, the great healing, the great freedom, the great creativity, the great efficiency and efficacy, the great intimacy and connection all hinge on which reality you're in. As I'll explain later, every word in the clinical vocabulary brings with it the entire clinical reality complete with its role/power relations. Every word brings with it a world. We speak things into existence. Never before has such importance been placed on the words we use and the subjectivity that produces those words.

All the therapeutic strategies and techniques are still valid. This is not antipsychiatry. This is a call for a transformation of the profession. The focus of professional education in mental health will be on relationship, language, dialogic skill, and a perspective of empowerment. Scott Miller calls therapy a craft; I call it an art. And, as pointed out in Miller et al.'s recent article (2013), training will be far more intimate because when you're dealing with the actions, attitudes, and feelings of a therapist you're really dealing with the therapist's subjectivity and vocabulary (of which mindfulness is only a part).

It is the convergence of these three lines of inquiry and research that has created the coherence, ripe for articulation, of a new paradigm in mental health. This is the purpose of this book.

II

The Linguistic Paradigm

FIVE

The Social Construction of Reality

Two thousand five hundred years ago Plato posited the foundations of Western philosophy; to put it simply: there are *appearances* and there is a *reality* behind those appearances; that our sensory perception is only an allusion to, an imperfect copy of, a corresponding eternal, perfect, and changeless reality. As Alfred North Whitehead (1929) once said, "The safest general characterization of the European philosophical tradition is that it consists of a series of footnotes to Plato." Not unlike psychiatric diagnoses, the concepts of the Western philosophical tradition (e.g., mind, matter, free will, justice, causality) were used as if they existed independently of human beings and that human beings discovered them along with their terminology. Philosophical knowledge consisted of analyzing these metaphysical concepts—as if anyone knew what these meant—in search of reality beyond appearances.

Two thousand three hundred years of philosophizing later, Friedrich Nietzsche concluded that we can dispense with the idea of a "reality" and that all we're left with is appearances—appearances shaped in language. This was the death of Western philosophy and birth of the postmodern worldview. As Nietzsche put it,

> Against that positivism which stops before phenomena, saying "there are only facts," I should say: no, it is precisely facts that do not exist, only interpretations. (Kaufman, 1976, 458)

The potential for relativism (all is permitted) and nihilism (no absolute truth means no meaning at all) was tempered by later American pragmatist and neopragmatist philosophers.

Notwithstanding the controversy of relativism or whether or not there's a "thing itself" behind all the appearances, the reality (appearances or perceptions) we all experience is extremely malleable—mirroring the plasticity of the brain. Different cultures employ language to carve out different realities such that the end result is our being better adapted to the environment in which we find ourselves. For example, the Laplanders of Norway, Sweden, and Finland have over 180 snow and ice related words as well as 1,000 words for reindeer (Robson, 2013).

There are no absolute truths—just more or less practical truths organized and handed down generationally in the form of culture. No particular culture holds privileged access to the truth. Culture, though not absolutely true in its conceptions, has its practical value.

Have you ever noticed how different cultures not only have different languages and practices but even different worldviews? Even within the same culture if we go back in time—imaginatively through historical novels or film—we see similar variability. So culture, indeed reality, changes historically as well as geographically. Moreover, each individual embodies her or his own culture differently. Having a culture means inhabiting a particular reality, a reality that comes into existence with both language and various practices. Language, culture, reality, and the human brain are all amazingly malleable. Yes, reality is malleable!

Culture is the human construction of reality; a social construction of reality. As infants the adults in our lives impress upon us language, values, and practices—that is, the reality *de jour*—intended to transform us from the instinct-driven infant into a person who can coordinate and integrate into the surrounding culture, society, and family. In the postmodern world we describe this as enculturation: the process of transformation from being dominated by primitive instincts to being in subjection to culture.

Peter L. Berger and Thomas Luckmann were sociologists in the 1960s whose seminal book, *The Social Construction of Reality* (1966), helped lay the foundation for social constructivists thinking in postmodernist philosophy. In their book they use a thought experiment to illustrate how realities are socially constructed:

> Imagine two survivors of some ecological disaster coming together to start a new society. Imagine that they are a man and a woman who come from very different cultures. Even if they share no language, no religion, and no presuppositions about how labor is to be divided, or what place work, play, communal ritual, and private contemplation have in a good society, if culture of any sort is to continue, they must begin to coordinate their activities. As they do this, some agreed-upon habits and distinctions will emerge: certain substances will be treated as food, certain places found or erected to serve as shelter, each will begin to assume certain routine daily tasks, and they will almost certainly develop a shared language. Between the two founding members of the emerging society, the habits and distinctions that arise will remain "tenuous, easily changeable, almost playful, even while they attain a measure of objectivity by the mere fact of their formation" (Berger and Luckmann, 1966, 58). They will always be able to remember,

> "This is how we decided to do this," or "It works better if I assume this role." They will carry some awareness that other possibilities exist. However, even in their generation, institutions such as "childcare," "farming," and "building" will have begun to emerge.
>
> For the children of the founding generation, "This is how we decided" will be more like "This is how it's done." Mothers and farmers and builders will be treated as always-having-existing types of people. The rough-and-ready procedures for building houses or planting crops that our original two survivors pieced together will be more-or-less codified as the rules for how to build a house or plant corn. In all likelihood laws will have been written about where, when, and how buildings may be built or crops may be planted. It is hard not to imagine that customs governing the proper rites for starting a family or harvesting a crop will have come to be, and that certain individuals will be identified as the proper people to perform those rites. Institutions like women's societies and masons' guilds will have begun to emerge.
>
> By the fourth generation of our imaginary society, "This is how it is done" will have become "This is the way the world is; this is reality." As Berger and Luckmann (1966, 60) put it, "An institutional world . . . is experienced as an objective reality." (Freedman and Combs, 1996, 22–23)

So we can see how conventional truths appear obvious only because we are born into institutions and traditions in which they are assumed true and spoken of accordingly.

Science is the apparent exception to this cultural relativity. Because of the rigor of its methods it appears to establish absolute truths that are objective and therefore transcend culture; whatever science says is "the truth." Time and relevance prohibit a discussion of the fallibility of science, but for our purposes, we can assume that what the latest science tells us we can assume as "true," at least provisionally.

Getting back to the Digital Statistical Manual (DSM). Because psychiatry claims to have its foundations in science, the assumption is its claims or "truths" (e.g., "diagnoses") can, more or less, be promoted with the authority of science behind them. But as was mentioned previously the only thing scientific about the DSM is that it uses statistics to come up with correlations and categories. And as we will see in later chapters, with repeated use the diagnostic label loses its status as an abstraction and becomes reified: made concrete or real. For something to be understood as a real physical entity, but unable to be physically observed (even with the aid of technology), is to posit a metaphysical entity. Notwithstanding the enormous problem that reification is, what if the best way to help someone is not to find out what category they fit in but quite the opposite, to explore their uniqueness, connect with it, and expand on it in the service of their unique commitments? We are effectively "blinded" by the label. As John Dewey (one of Carl Rogers's strong influences) in his *Human Nature and Conduct* (1922) explains:

> To classify is, indeed, as useful as it is natural. The indefinite multitude of particular and changing events is met by the mind with acts of defining, inventorying, and listing, reducing to common heads and tying up in bunches. . . . But when we assume that our lists and bunches represent fixed separations and collections in rerum natura [nature], we obstruct rather than aid our transactions with things. We are guilty of a presumption which nature promptly punishes. We are rendered incompetent to deal effectively with the delicacies and novelties of nature and life. . . . The tendency to forget the office of distinctions and classifications, and *to take them as marking things in themselves* is the current fallacy of scientific specialism. (131, my italics added)

In other words, reification of psychiatric labels renders us "incompetent to deal effectively with the delicacies and novelties" of our client's subjectivity. Yes, the DSM diagnoses with their reality status blind us to the most relevant and, otherwise salient, aspects of the person who comes for help: their nuanced interpretations of themselves and their world, their preferences, their concerns, their priorities, their strengths, their multifaceted natures, their conflicts, their non-verbal behavior, their responses to us—in a phrase, their worldview. A person's worldview and their response to us guide us in our moment-to-moment transactions in postmodern coaching. This is feedback-informed practice in real time.

Psychological theories and orientations (modalities) are almost by definition reifications as they act as organizing templates or interpretive lenses with which to selectively view a client and his/her relationships to the exclusion of all else about a client. Through repetition in the form of writing, speaking, and acting they are viewed as essential or absolute realities. William O'Hanlon uses an analogy of making holiday cookies to illustrate what happens when a theoretical template is imposed on a client (O'Hanlon and Wiener-Davis, 1989). Before coming to therapy a client's experience of themselves and their circumstances (or "the problem") is rather ambiguous, undefined, malleable. It's like cookie dough. The amorphous blob of cookie dough is forced through the cookie press (a tube, funnel, and mold pressed against a baking pan) and, conforming to the mold at the tip, it becomes a star, Santa Clause, or Christmas tree. Similarly, the client's experience and problem get "molded" as the therapist selectively views, responds, and communicates—as the absolute, objective, or scientific truth of "what's going on"—through his/her vocabulary. A client after contact with a cognitive behavioral therapist will "have" cognitive distortions as his/her problem. This same client with a psychodynamic therapist will leave the session with unresolved childhood conflicts. Speaking with a diagnostically minded therapist would leave this same client thinking they have a "mental illness" ("bipolar disorder," "depression," "obsessive compulsive disorder," "borderline personality disorder") complete with "chemical imbalance," life-long duration, and a life-long need to comply with a treatment regimen. This same client would leave the Jungian therapist's office with archetypes and a collective unconscious. Like baking cookies, repeated contact with the "heat" of the theoretical lens causes what would otherwise be an interpretation to "harden" or reify (make real as an objective truth). O'Hanlon's point is that if language creates "the problem," then why don't we use language to create an easy-to-solve problem! In her groundbreaking book, *Conversation, Language, and Possibilities*, Harlene Anderson (1997) adds:

> What seems to be an identifiable objective reality—a problem—is only a product of descriptions, the product of social construction. (73)

Another example is Sigmund Freud's idea of ego, superego, and id. As original and profound as Freud's work was he believed that his work was scientific and that the ego, superego, and id existed as real objective (albeit non-physical) entities. In other words, that he "discovered" them as causes of the observable human experience and behavior, when in fact he made distinctions in language which, in effect, created them. The amorphous unity of "the world" can be carved in many ways with words, none of which can lay claim to essential or absolute truth to the exclusion of the others. Exactly like "psychiatric diagnoses" and "chemical imbalance," though no one has ever seen an ego, superego, or id nor their neural correlates they're still spoken of as "things" that cause real-world observable behaviors. This is a form of metaphysics. Mental health professionals inhabit this psychologistic subjectivity. As Søren Kierkegaard (1846/1992) proclaimed, "Subjectivity is truth." In other words, it appears as truth, it appears as reality. As hyperbole it emphasizes how hard it is to get a handle on.

Institutional, conventional, and cultural truths are maintained simply in their being spoken. In his provocative book *Did the Greeks Believe Their Myths: An Essay on the Constitutive Imagination*, Paul Veyne (1988)—borrowing on the work of Michel Foucault—described how cultural beliefs are maintained through convention and speaking. In other words, because the Greeks *customarily* spoke of the gods—and the narratives in which the Greek gods were embedded—the imagined "Greek god" worldview was maintained; maintained not as in interesting speculation, but as an obvious truth of human existence. In fact, the Greeks often attributed their irrational, passion-driven, impulsive, and often-destructive actions to them being impelled by the gods—much like the irrational feelings-thoughts-behaviors of today's people are attributed to the "chemical imbalance" or "psychiatric diagnosis." In both cases, metaphorically, imaginatively, conventionally, and ritually constituted worldviews were/are used for their explanatory power, each prescribing their respective solutions: animal sacrifice and psychotropic "balancing" medications. I wish this were where the similarity ended. As we will see in chapter 8 ("Why This Is the Wrong Metaphor to Begin With") where we cover the power of belief in one investigation as much as 80 percent of the effect of antidepressant medications was placebo effect (Kirsch, 2002). So be it myth, belief, superstition, suggestion, expectation, or political discourse, advertising, or professional rhetoric there's much power in it; but as it was with the ancient Greeks it keeps us from further innovation, be it in the form of science or art (in this case language).

So in other words, the everyday language (manifested in ideas, beliefs, values, ways of living, and practices) we use is not describing an "objective reality" outside of us; but, instead, it is creating a subjective—albeit consensual—reality. Liberal democracy has greatly facilitated cultural evolution. Things are "true" and "good" because enough people say so (the manipulation of public opinion by those in power aside). As of this writing cultural pluralism, diversity, gay marriage, the right to sexual orientation, the right to gender identity, the legalization of marijuana, and immigrant rights are all salient issues that are changing our cultural landscape in the West. As we've noted professional vocabularies speak and write consensual realities into existence—in our case psychiatry/psychology. The clinical world where "patients" suffer from "mental illness," "diagnoses," "chemical imbalances" and are in need of "treatment" is a fabrication, not objective reality. A fabrication with devastating consequences to the individual, society, and civilization as we will see in part III ("A Fundamental Egalitarianism").

To summarize: The entire psychiatric and psychological vocabularies and worldviews do not speak with the authority of science and, consequently, the realities that these institutions/professions promulgate is quite arbitrary; their "truths" are cultural artifacts rather than scientific realities. And, like other cultural realities, they're usually manipulated by powerful interests (read: the pharmaceutical industry). I recommend *Saving Normal: An Insider's Revolt against Out-of-Control Psychiatric Diagnosis, DSM-5, Big Pharma, and the Medicalization of Ordinary Life* by Allen Frances (2013a), former chairperson for the DSM-IV. Furthermore, these purported realities are spoken into existence; once you stop speaking that language they stop existing!

Moreover, and most importantly, as we will see in chapter 8 (on metaphors), the application of traditional (reductive) science to human behavior and the human spirit was a mistake, a mistake commonly referred to as *scientism*. We need neuroscience, neuroplasticity, and complexity theory to support our language and practices in helping people discover and live their preferred life.

THE NATURE OF LANGUAGE SYSTEMS—ONE WORD BRINGS WITH IT A WORLD

Words don't lead isolated existences. Words evolve out of established networks of other words we refer to as contexts or vocabularies. Any given word brings with it the entire context in which it's embedded. *As such with any given word we experience a reality, a world.* As I wrote in my 2006 paper "The Social Construction of Mental Illness and Its Implications for the Recovery Model":

> When we speak as if someone has a diagnosis or has a "mental illness" we are unwittingly creating a reality—a reality in which human beings are transformed into the "mentally ill." When we use words such as "mental illness," "schizophrenia," "symptoms," "tangential speech," "clinical this or that," "treatment plan," "assessment"—we are unwittingly bringing forth the entire context, the hierarchical and paternalistic role relationship together with the sticky morass of pathological and deficit-based perspectives. Jill Freedman and Gene Combs (1996) write:
>
> Speaking isn't neutral or passive. Every time we speak, we bring forth a reality. Each time we share words we give legitimacy to the distinctions that those words bring forth (29).
>
> Words, abstractions, theories, and beliefs focus our attention. Heinz von Foerster (1984), the famous cybernetician and constructivist, concluded: "Believing is seeing." We "see" those behaviors that confirm the diagnosis and hardly notice those behaviors that don't. Because those are the behaviors noticed and responded to, the client experiences herself defined as such, and, by way of self-fulfilling prophecy, feels a strong "relational pull" to behave accordingly. It doesn't take an advanced knowledge of systems theory or cybernetics to see how we amplify the "symptoms" and reify (make real) the "labels" by the use of the pathologizing language. The irony and tragedy is profound. (Walker, 2006)

The world or reality we inhabit is vocabularically realized. In the postmodern world we typically refer to contexts (even science) as vocabularies or narratives to divest them of any absolute or essential truth status. The term "vocabulary" includes words, concepts, presuppositions, beliefs, as well as the associated actions and practices.

As we mentioned earlier, from a historical perspective, the current vocabulary or narrative of mental health has its origins in the disease model, which has its beginnings in the reductionistic and mechanistic models of the Enlightenment. The clinical model of mental health was a love grandchild of humanity's love affair with reason. We now realize that when studying complex systems reason and reductive science are insufficient. We need a new vocabulary that takes into account the power of language and neuroplasticity.

In the language paradigm we understand that the possibility and power of human transformation lies in language. This is all but obvious when we look at the phenomenon of culture.

Understanding culture and language is our clue as to how the brain as a complex system changes. The interpersonal pressure of culture (through the force and repetition of language) takes what would otherwise be a feral animal and transforms it into a person. The domains of personal and spiritual growth and development could be seen as meta-culture as we consciously strive to use language to help us deal with our default enculturation and animal instincts, perform better in the world, and achieve a more satisfying subjectively felt experience. Though the terms "culture" and "subjectivity" are roughly synonymous, when we focus on the changeability of whatever this phenomenon is we refer to it as subjectivity. The vocabulary of human transformation reveals the reality of the pliability of human subjectivity and the malleability of the human brain.

Furthermore the modernist world is unaware of the power of language because its systems of vocabularies (e.g., disciplines) are self-affirming, self-enclosed realities. What we postmodernists would call their language systems (or games), modernists would call established truth or objective reality. Because a world comes into existence with language, we don't see the framework of language behind the manifest world, we just see a world. This effect was so startling to Martin Heidegger that he claimed that *we don't use language, language uses us*. Consequently, the scaffolding of language concealed, our actions are perfectly and reflexively in accord with this world that simply shows up as a result of our exposure to a vocabulary.

Said simply, believing and seeing are mutually reinforcing—believing is seeing and seeing is believing. We see only that which confirms the belief. Thus *hermeneutically sealed* (interpretively closed) it is very, very difficult to escape our self-affirming reality. One's own institutionalization is very hard to see. The entire profession needs to take its own advice, needs to transcend its own fixed and self-defeating beliefs and practices. We owe a great debt of gratitude to the postmodern thinkers who through their historical and literary investigations revealed how words create realities more than they describe or represent them.

The practical implications of this are enormous. We have to throw out the entire deficit-based, pathologizing, and institutionalizing vocabulary! We have to dispense with the entire clinical rhetoric! The entire clinical reality is brought forth with any given word. Programs often superficially layer "recovery," "client-driven," "wellness," "strength-based" approaches on top of the "rock hard" clinical *reality* of pathology and deficit focus; the result, a kind of odd, internally inconsistent chimera. In other words, these putatively client-self-determining programs are still steeped in the vocabulary that supports the psychologistic, paternalistic power relations and still have the problem of domination/submission, colonialization, marginalization—all of which are invisible to the participants involved.

In its place we will create a new language of empowerment drawing from past human wisdom and humanity's evolving transcendent vocabulary. And, yes, to avoid the chimera above, vocabularic consistency is the key. Through a kind of language-immersion process vocabulary, practice, and felt experience become consistent and need stay consistent in order for a culture of empowerment to come into existence and be maintained.

The vocabularies, perspectives, and practices of personal growth and spiritual transformation are already in-the-world. Postmodern coaching involves an egalitarian relationship structure that allows for the integration of a client's current worldview with that of this more evolved frame of reference, all in the service of the commitment we have to the quality of our lives. We simply tailor-make tools—as opposed to a one-size-fits-all approach—to help people achieve their objectives.

Furthermore, the cash can still flow in the appropriate directions without the clinical realities and categories. In my experience medical necessity can be documented and government benefits can be established by using a normative perspective (what is a client unable to do that most people can do) and descriptive language.

DIFFERENT WORDS = DIFFERENT CONTEXTS

When we say "medications" the entire pathologizing clinical reality, complete with subjugating roles, comes into existence. The word "medication" brings forth the entire medication-chemical-imbalance-centered universe and the passive, insecure, dependent "patient." In contrast, when we say "pills" we defy the pathologizing context and assert the context of empowerment. The word "pill" means that it is one tool among many and that we are each individually responsible for how we feel and how our life turns out. When pressed to say what would otherwise be called a "diagnosis" I say "mental health code" or "label" instead of "diagnosis." Tongue-in-cheek, "medicine person" instead of "psychiatrist." "Person" instead of "patient." "Being stuck" instead of "having depression." Calling the "waiting room" a "lobby" is part of the shift. Where "assessments" are still popular, you could say "gathering background information required by the current system."

In the beginning this may seem like unnecessary "hair splitting" or an issue of political correctness, but eventually, through enough deliberate practice, the power of language, context, and of a single word becomes evident. In the beginning it may seem totally impractical; yet I've maintained this reality in an orthodox mental health institutional setting for the past twenty-five years. The amazing results will speak for themselves, despite your unorthodox way of speaking. As we will see in chapter 14 on "guerilla tactics," realizing the postmodern worldview in a modernist institutional framework is an art form in itself.

Like the ancient Greeks, as long as we keep speaking the metaphysical constructions into existence (be they "gods" or "psychiatric diagnoses")—by using the words themselves or any of the words in their context—they continue to have life-determining consequences. I once had a client say to me, "I take Adderall for my ADHD [attention deficit/hyperactivity disorder]." I responded back, "So you take Adderall because it helps you concentrate." These two sentences are *paradigms apart*; they represent the difference between the worldview of the patient versus the worldview of the person.

THE PARADOX OF REALITY AND INTERPRETATION

When I say reality is socially constructed, I don't mean to imply that there is no "reality" to "reality," that we can create any reality we want by means of language and interpretation. The question of whether or not I could be an NBA player at this point in my life has realistic considerations, which would be foolish to ignore—I can't speak this into existence. On the other hand, Nietzsche claims (paraphrasing), "There are no facts, only interpretations." Yet, is a rock falling on your foot a matter of interpretation? Is there a reality to the rock independent of language and interpretation? If there's no "thing in itself" (à la Friedrich Nietzsche), or we cannot know it independent of interpretation (à la Immanuel Kant), why does it hurt so much?

As the philosophers of the Scottish commonsense realism, to which we are heir, were to say, common sense has a reality all its own. The cold and rugged terrain of Scotland would not yield to be reinterpreted other than cold and rugged. In a kind of reactionary response to Kant's Copernican revolution (i.e., we know the world by projecting space, time, causality, substance onto it) and Nietzsche's nihilism (or perspectivism), the Scottish commonsense philosophers insisted sense data, causality, substance, space, time, and, finally, morality were all to be taken as objective facts (thus the idea of "self-evident truth"). In other words, our minds don't construct "facts," they simply recognize them (as they would otherwise exist in the world even if humans didn't exist)—thus establishing human beings back at their rightful place at the center of the universe. This was a big shot in the arm for the *consensual* basis of truth.

The realism of the Scottish commonsense philosophy prevailed in our socioeconomic-political American landscape in the form of the *self-evident truths* supporting liberal democracy and capitalism; and to this we can be eternally grateful. Furthermore, this is part of the rationalist (including mechanistic and reductionistic) frame of reference that has structured our lives—and our minds—in the West. In the United States the very profound, though esoteric, and *seemingly* useless insights of existential and postmodern Europe were to yield to the practical expediency of the political economy.

We speak of being realistic for practical purposes. Though he was quite justified, we need not go so far as Ernst Cassirer (1963) in saying that even sensory experience is a function of language and interpretation. Yet much of the world of objects and events legitimately yields to multiple interpretations (or multiple descriptions). So our criteria for choosing between interpretations become efficacy, utility, efficiency, and in many cases, morality. Realism itself is a point of view.

In the world in general and in medicine in particular realism translates into how well our words "map nature." In other words, how well do our words (e.g., diagnoses) correspond to the world of physical objects. For example, a broken bone is a physical object that can be assessed, diagnosed, and treated. The diagnosis of *broken bone* "maps nature" because we can operate or x-ray and see a physical structure we call a "bone" divided in a way we call "broken"; which explains the symptoms of pain, immobility, etc., that we observe.

However when we're talking about psychiatric diagnoses and "chemical imbalances" we're talking about failure from the perspective of both *realism* and *utility*. As we will see in chapter 7 ("The DSM Criticized by Its Makers") when it comes to psychiatric diagnoses they are not real even by the standards of realism. As noted by the creators of the DSM themselves, *psychiatric diagnoses do not map nature*, there are no characteristic neural correlates that they correspond to. In the lead up to the DSM-5, Steven Hyman, member of the DSM-5 Task Force and chair of the International Advisory Group on the Revision of ICD-10 (International Statistical Classification of Diseases, 10th ed.), admits:

> Overall, there is evidence that the current diagnoses and their corresponding sets of criteria fall short of mapping nature. . . . Owing to the limited understanding of the biological underpinnings of mental disorders that neuroscience and genetics could provide at the time, the diagnoses within the DSM-III and the DSM-IV have necessarily been based on clinical observation. Despite the optimism of Robins and Guze, laboratory tests for the major, common psychiatric disorders have not yet materialized. (2007, 727)

In the words of Allen Frances, MD, chair of the DSM-IV Task Force and author of *Saving Normal: An Insider's Revolt against Out-of-Control Psychiatric Diagnosis, DSM-5, Big Pharma, and the Medicalization of Ordinary Life*:

> The expectation that there would be a simple gene or neurotransmitter or circuitry explanation for any mental disorder has turned out to be naïve and illusory. (2013a, 10)

So by the criteria of realism psychiatric diagnoses and their "chemical imbalance" counterpart fail miserably. We'll talk more of this later.

As we've seen in the previous chapter on neuroplasticity and will see in chapter 8 ("Why This Is the Wrong Metaphor to Begin With") complexity neuroscience's consideration of the brain (1) as a whole, (2) in its adaptive capabilities, and (3) in its social context gives us a more accurate map or metaphor of nature. The physical brain as a whole has neural structures, systems, tissues that correspond *not* to static "chemical imbalances" and "psychiatric diagnoses," but instead to changing neuronal patterns (neuroplasticity) that reflect the human brain's reflexive relationship with thinking, language, behavior, and the environment. From a realistic perspective neuroplasticity is a fact, and it correlates to real-world physical observation (with sophisticated equipment) and concrete behavior change as we saw earlier.

Alas, the search for the Holy Grail continues both in reductive neuroscience and precision medicine. But even if they're able to scrape together some kind of evidence of neural correlates to some diagnoses, some of the time, complexity neuroscience, epigenetics, and the postmodern linguistic paradigm make this irrelevant. In complex systems, such as the human brain, the parts interact in a way that produces emergent properties of the whole that, in turn, feedback to alter the parts. The human brain like other complex systems is irreducible: the emergent properties of the whole (language, thinking, subjectivity, behavior) cannot be understood by an analysis of the parts (neurons, synapses, and neurotransmitters). Much like the wetness of water cannot be studied by an analysis of the separate elements hydrogen and oxygen.

Consciousness is an emergent property of the physical human brain. And, as we've seen, interpretation is integral to consciousness. Higher, broader, and more profound levels of interpretation contextualize lower levels; in other words we are capable of resubjectifying ourselves—to use the vernacular, one can become a bigger person. The human brain is malleable and, not surprisingly, human subjectivity is malleable. Our lower self-realizations may (or may not) always be a propensity, however, with coaching and practice, far from *destiny*. To label a tendency is to make it your destiny.

The problem with unwarranted realism—or hardening of the categories—is that it reifies in places where interpretive flexibility would vastly better serve us. We can interpret and reinterpret, describe and redescribe until we get better and better results. This is a basic tenant of neopragmatism. Human subjective suffering and practical struggle is a reality; but to label it an illness is a construction.

A compromise between realism and perspectivism might be that concrete particulars do exist, but abstractions don't. Have you ever seen a "dog"? No, you've seen a particular dog (or many particular dogs), not a dog as an abstraction. "Mental illness," "psychiatric diagnoses," and "psychiatric symptoms" are abstractions or social constructions; but individually experienced emotional pain and various counterproductive behaviors do exist. Once we call a behavior a "symptom" we've made a very big and unnecessary interpretive leap into the "clinical world." As people get a more powerful perspective on life and begin taking constructive action the counterproductive behaviors and emotional suffering are shed like a snake's skin—i.e., the so-called "symptoms" are handled indirectly.

At this point I want to express my gratitude to Allen Frances, for his brilliance of insight and boldness of action in his attempt to Save Normal. Yet, at the same time, Dr. Frances is exemplary of so many contemporary thinkers who while pointing in the right direction have pushed up against the modernist ceiling only to *intimate* the light of possibility that is the postmodern linguistic breakthrough. He relates:

> The best way to understand the essence of mental disorder—what it is and what it is not—is to compare the balls and strikes calls of three different umpires. Most of epistemology boils down to their competing opinions on how well we can ever apprehend reality.
>
> Umpire One: "There are balls and there are strikes and I call them as they are."
> Umpire Two: "There are balls and there are strikes and I call them as I see them."
> Umpire Three: "There are no balls and there are no strikes until I call them."
>
> Umpire One believes that mental disorders are real "diseases";
> Umpire Three that they are fanciful "myths";
> Umpire Two that they are something between—useful constructs and provide no more (but no less) than a *best current guess on how to sort psychiatric distress*. (2013a, 18; my italics)

"Sort psychiatric distress"! What on earth for? Statistical sorting and labeling have got nothing to do with human change and transformation. On the contrary, to label a propensity is to ensure its destiny. Would the best way to help people abide by the law be to label those transgressors as criminals and make fine distinctions and gradations as to different kinds of criminals? Or similarly with children with problematic behavior? Does commonsense human wisdom have a chance against our theoretical ontology, our Laputan compulsion to classify at the expense of the universe of human transformation and possibility available to us? Is earth the insane asylum as George Bernard Shaw declaimed?

Field guides should be restricted to bird watching! The days of "neutral," "clinical" observation of people are long gone, to be replaced by subject-to-subject real-time participation! Anyone cognizant of the power of language knows "sorting" and labeling inevitably leads to reification and reification is the last thing you want to do if you're interested in change. Educate people how change occurs, don't delude them into thinking abstractions are real in-the-world entities. Make distinctions that perpetuate change!

We abandoned Kant and postmodern Europe at great cost. With great scientific, technological, economic, political, social, and military success in the West came great hubris. Excessive pride led to a misidentification of its culture with absolute truth. Consequently the West lost its ability to self-reflect, to be self-critical. Ironically, given what it purports to do for the individual, the mental health profession suffers from this same solipsism.

We can admit Nietzsche was famous for hyperbole, exaggerating to make a point. But when it comes to the human brain and human subjectivity he was right on. With due respect to realism, the power of thinking, feeling, and language have yet to be tapped into. Language, expectations, presuppositions, connotations, declaration, assertion, role positioning all have powerful creative or, if not careful, destructive potential. Because of a bad track record, there may be no realistic basis to ask a client, "What will you be doing when you're feeling better?" But it works a lot better than asking, "What would you be doing if you got over this depression?" By answering the first question ("What will s/he be doing?) the client affirms the presupposition embedded in the question that they will be feeling better. As is well known with experimental classroom studies with children, expectations and presuppositions have enormous power. After all what do you think the placebo effect is!

Thus we conclude that psychiatric diagnoses and the clinical worldview in general fail with respect to both realism (or the correspondence theory of truth, or mapping of nature) and utility (the pragmatic/perspectivist theory of truth). To be continued in chapter 7, "The DSM Criticized by Its Makers."

SIX

Vocabularies, Institutionalization, and Power

Words, concepts, vocabularies frame our experience and determine our actions, thoughts, and feelings. Moreover, like water is to the fish, we just plain live in vocabularies; we don't see them, yet they determine us. Postmodernists use terms like "vocabulary" or "narrative" to indicate the absence of absolute or essential truth. In the modernist world we "swim around" in a vocabulary thinking it is objective reality. This holds true for both the professional vocabularies in mental health as well as the institutional vocabularies (private or state run) of the agencies that employ mental health professionals. And, if words weren't amazing enough already they also define power relations.

THE PSYCHOLOGISTIC VOCABULARY

Before the postmodern breakthrough, the world we inhabit was seen as obviously true. For a long time Western culture was deemed the truth in comparison with other cultures. Through the process of enculturation and education all sorts of cultural, institutional, and professional beliefs are handed down as obvious truths. Professionals in psychiatry and psychology experience their concepts and corresponding practices as objective truth—obviously true. For a colleague to question their truths—from their frame of reference—would be a sign of a lack of professional education, unprofessional conduct, rebelliousness, antipsychiatricness, or the like.

Postmodernism changed all this in a very profound way. Furthermore, because the harder to arrive at philosophical frameworks filter down slowly to the culture as a whole, few are aware of this. So we stand at the dawning of a new postmodern age, but it must be worked into, spoken, written about, acted on, and practiced in order to prevail against the currents of the prevailing modernist cultural discourses.

From the postmodern perspective all the obvious truths of psychology are transformed into or seen as a perspective or point of view that is vocabularically constituted—made of words and concepts. The word "vocabulary" deconstructs the truth status of any particular interpretive framework. This might be contrasted, for example, with the word "theory." Where theory implies that there is some essential and absolute truth to be discovered and that a theory is an educated guess at that truth; vocabulary implies that there is no such truth and that words are tools for living. The clinical vocabulary's (medical model's) pseudo-link with science does not exempt it from being a cultural artifact, i.e., being one vocabulary among others. So now vocabularies can be evaluated with regard to their utility or consequences.

The psychologistic vocabulary has been viewed from the modernist world as absolute or objective truth. Professionals and lay people alike utter sentences that presuppose the existence of psychologistic concepts or entities. "We need more resources to treat the homeless mentally ill." "Does psychotherapy work with bipolar disorder?" "Does depression run in your family?" "We need to fight the stigma of mental illness." "If I hear voices, does that mean I have schizophrenia?" Such seeming benign expressions are the vehicles for pernicious presuppositions. While being occupied with the content of the sentence/question (e.g., the response, "There are cognitive therapies that work with bipolar disorder.") we're oblivious to the presuppositions embedded in the context whose reality is perpetuated merely by virtue of uttering the sentence/question and someone else responding to the content. Any way you answer the question, "When did you stop beating your wife?" you affirm the presupposition that you beat your wife. Furthermore, as was revealed in chapter 5, any term from the clinical vocabulary ("treatment plan," "assessment," "peers," "recovery," etc.) brings forth the reality status of all the other terms, including "mental illness" and "diagnoses."

When it comes to "education" and "training," with enough exposure to the vocabulary and practices, the young student emerges into a clinical world. This world, authorized by those in power, is consensually, conversationally, and conventionally (including in writing) maintained. Forgetful of having made it up, superstitiously prone human beings see their culture (in this case a kind of subculture) as an obvious and unmediated reality.

Recognizing psychiatry as a vocabulary, one of many vocabularies, we are now in a position to critically evaluate it. Absent this postmodern perspective, psychology as an obvious truth has a built-in explanatory system that explains its failures and hides its consequences—it's hermeneutically sealed (i.e., it is a closed and self-affirming system of interpretation). Among the explanations: "That client is not ready to change," "She lacks motivation," "Mental illness is permanent; you just learn to live with it." The client's "resistance," "lack of motivation," "non-compliance," "unwillingness to keep appointments," or "chemical imbalance" are the clinician's wild card to explain away therapeutic failures and in the process avoid taking responsibility for acquiring new skills and perspectives that might have otherwise made the difference. For example, what could I have done differently to support my client in making his appointments? Perhaps he wasn't engaged. What could I have done to better engage him? Instead, the client's therapy-unfriendly behavior is explained as a mental illness-related or non-mental-illness-related trait of the client; and the professional is off the hook and left helpless.

It should be no surprise that the development and advancement of the profession as a whole has been outpaced by the pre-global warming glaciers. At best the artful and experimental process of determining what works in psychotherapy, of indeed learning from experience, is dramatically circumscribed within the range of theoretical categories, options, explanations, and interventions available. At its worst, and unfortunately the rule and not the exception, the client is the convenient scapegoat for "therapeutic" failures and nothing is learned. And, yes, to repeat, I'm saying to take responsibility for therapeutic outcome is to never involve the client in our explanation of failure, but to engage the inquiry of what we could have done differently.

The nature of vocabularies is such that you need a postmodern vantage point outside a particular vocabulary in order to critically evaluate it as a vocabulary (or perspective) and not absolute/obviously true. Once indoctrinated into an institutional vocabulary the rivalry begins in the knowledge/power game. Moreover the higher up in the pecking order you are in this hierarchy of "knowledge" the more you're invested in maintaining this reality.

Because of the way words and ideas "travel" many psychologistic terms and ideas have filtered "down" (or "up" depending on your point of view) to the mainstream culture. "Dysfunctional family," "bipolar," "depression," "issues," "psychotic," "addiction" are but a few. Again, since society in general is in its infancy when it comes to what it means to be in a relationship and how to effectively manage relationships, following the lead of the mental health profession, we resort to labeling. And, needless to say, these labels are toxic to the relationship, both professional and personal—this will be addressed in the last section in this chapter: "Labeling Is Lethal to Relationships."

THE SPECTER OF INSTITUTIONALIZATION

Many mental health services take place in large institutions like hospitals and community mental health clinics. In addition to the professional vocabulary, with these institutions we have an institutional vocabulary to reckon with. Professionals are unable to see their own institutionalization that complements and supports the easily recognizable institutionalization of their clients.

"We need to assess that acute client for our FSP program," "We provide services for service area 12, for people outside of our catchment area we refer to CDP." "She is a meds-only client." "We need to contact the hospital in order to coordinate care." "Mom [referring to the mother of children detained by child services] denies using drugs, but we're mandating random drug testing." The term "services" is a staple of institutionalizing rhetoric. Typically, statements like these seem like harmless communications or statements of fact. Indeed, within the institutional context, to recite institutional rhetoric is a sign of professional competence. However, to the person cognizant of the power of language and context, they are far more than simple communications.

Every communication has content and command aspect (Jackson, 1965) and it is the command or role-enforcing aspect that clients feel and that positions them in the clinical realm as incompetent, fragile, a "good client," uncooperative, non-compliant, compliant, untrustworthy, "mentally ill," or otherwise "broken" and in the institutional realm as a "patient," something to be "processed," a "manipulator," a "malingerer," someone "working" the system, or a source of revenue or liability.

When it comes to human relationships connotations are more important that denotations. Remember that the nature of the therapeutic relationship is a "felt" experience. The command aspect of communication is a "felt" experience; we feel a "pull" to be a certain way. We're being scripted. In the land where "compliance" is the supreme value, the role positioning that occurs in professional and institutional vocabularies is closer to parent-child than adult-to-adult; and this is definitely a felt experience, that of subjection. Recall that it is the quality of the consciously or unconsciously felt (right brain to right brain) experience that is the basis of attunement, intersubjectivity, the relationship, and the alliance—the firmly established essential factors in the success of psychotherapy.

Institutional procedure, protocol, and rhetoric are designed for the handling and "processing" (words normally reserved for objects) of mass numbers of people. It's no small thing when someone states, "I *feel* like a number." It's important to remember that institutionalization is an aspect of a therapist's, psychiatrist's, and other ancillary (e.g., administrative) staff's subjectivities; as such it is not at all obvious. But once you see it, you see how pervasive and insidious it is, and furthermore, you become aware that no one else is aware of it. It is clear as daylight in their actions as well as in their words, phrases, and sentences. Subjectivity is revealed in behavior and communication (both verbal and non-verbal). From this postmodern realm people's subjectivity is broadcasting loud and clear despite them not having a clue to its existence. Unfortunately, the people we're supposed to be helping appear as "cogs" or "numbers" or "patients" simply by virtue of the routine rhetoric of the institution.

Over the past twenty years there has been a movement in the corporate world to try to personalize customer service—perhaps an attempt at "building relationships." Of course, scripted. After the 2007 banking crisis Citibank employees at my branch suddenly became my best friends. Almost universally in the corporate world customer service agents are mechanically empathetic. In a very programmed way they're required to ask you "how your day is going" and then proceed to robotically paraphrase back to you your problem and then communicate "how frustrating that must be." An institutionalized answer to the problem of institutionalization.

Institutional rhetoric creates an institutional identity where the speaker becomes an instrument of the institution. From this frame of reference clients are expected—like cogs in a giant machine—to conform to the logic and policy of the institution, that is, to become passive and compliant patients. Institutionalization is objectification of persons.

When we learn and embody the vocabulary, interpretations, presuppositions, and practices of an institution (which is a kind of culture) we, to varying degrees, leave our personhood behind and become institutional agents. As we will see in chapter 10 people vary in their capacity to identify with roles. The problem is with the phenomenon of identification. Unbeknownst to us, like out of some science fiction film, the moment we arrive on the "set," in some unconscious way, the role takes over, we become the role. Not surprisingly, people who become their roles tend to rise quickly in the corporate or political arenas.

Institutional policies, programs, and procedures are routinized in employee practice and rhetoric, all of which comprises an institutional culture. Like cultural conformity in general, professional practice and rhetoric is enforced—when present rewarded with respect and admiration, when absent punished with overt or covert (the "gaze") ridicule or shame. Recall from Michel Foucault that "expert knowledge is power" and situates us hierarchically within a profession and/or an institution. Moreover, part of our invisible European heritage is that civility—in our case also professional competence—is conflated with deference to hierarchy.

The problem is that when people become instruments of institutions they see through the rhetoric, practices, and policies of the institution. The human element is lost. Clients are made objects and seen through the Procrustean bed of the rhetoric of the institution. Interfacing with "hollow" women and men (a reference to T. S. Eliot's 1925 poem[1])—that is, those identified with their institutional roles—is not so bad if you're trying to get your cable TV bill corrected. But when confronted with a human body that is an instrument of an institution, essentially demanding conformity, our clients are jammed further in their heads. This is true whether we're talking about a receptionist or psychologist. Whether performing an "assessment" or "empathy" (note the irony of "performing empathy") the net effect of the professional role is the same: just one more frustrating confrontation with the modern alienating world. Max Weber described the "mechanized petrification" of the human instruments of the Western bureaucratic institutions in his famous work *The Protestant Ethic and the Spirit of Capitalism* (1905/2001):

> Specialist without spirit, sensualist without heart; this nullity imagines that it has attained a level of humanity (Menschentums) never before achieved. (124)

The vast majority of people who seek mental health assistance need an authentic, compassionate, non-judgmental human-to-human encounter. To be authentic while having an organized, meaningful, and purposeful framework guiding a collaborative journey into intersubjective space, the final frontier, is an art form highly dependent on a therapist subjectivity that will support it.

The entire vocabulary of the institution reflects the bureaucratization of the modern self that Max Weber warned of. The bureaucratic organization of activities extends into roles and identities; we became cogs in institutions. Frank W. Elwell (2013) describes Weber's view of how technocratic thinking—the vocabulary, logic, and practices of an institution—have a pervasive effect on us:

> Weber's rationalization theory is that modernity promotes the growing dominance of technocratic thinking at the expense of critical thinking; as bureaucracy comes to dominate modern society, it becomes the dominant motivating force—*a mode of thought that becomes part of our very being*. (148; my italics added)

Yes, "part of our very being," and, as such, it's transparent to us; we can't see it.

Weber claimed that though bureaucratic institutions were essential for the coordination of activities in democratic political economies, they were notoriously inept at dealing with individual peculiarities. And what is a system of mental health if not dealing with individual peculiarities! Let me give a simple example. In my twenty-five plus years working in institutional mental health settings I've seen clients "blamed for" their inability to play by institutional rules; to take a simple example, when clients come late to or miss appointments (thus violating institutional policy). On one hand, the "strict" therapist—out to teach a lesson (thus not "enable" the client)—will insist on the client feeling the consequences of their behavior. On the other hand, the "pathologizing" therapist will see being late or missing appointments as symptoms of client's "mental disorder." These two styles of approach apply to a multitude of client behaviors that lie outside the institutional grid.

Moreover since *some* clients are able to modify their behavior in accordance with institutional demands, many staff view *all* clients as capable. Clients that are unable to "comply" are seen as troublemakers, manipulators, and otherwise irresponsible, deserving of institutional and policy consequences.

The issue is that people don't come to mental health institutions to learn how to be on time, to sit quietly in a waiting room, "comply" with "treatment," or any other normative expectation. They come to feel better and/or in some way achieve an important goal. In postmodern coaching we're passionate about helping people develop and achieve their passions. In this context a client's behavior is "good" or "bad" only in reference to their objectives.

Institutionalization is a manifestation of subjectivity. A person's subjectivity (or worldview) is revealed in his/her verbal and non-verbal language. Their feelings, thoughts, beliefs, and perspectives are all reflected in their words, sentences, inflections, and intonations. The body in its verbal and non-verbal behavior is a reflection of subjectivity. The subjectivity of the institutionalized professional or administrator represents a force imposed on the person seeking help. This is nothing more than the "blind" cultural transmission of values and practices. This sets up a role relationship of submission, more popularly referred to as "compliance." We're not here to "hold people accountable," we're here to help people reach their goals and occasionally to *act as liaisons* with some of the unyielding demands of our society or unavoidable institutional operating policies. When we represent institutional limitations ("If you're not on time we will have to reschedule you.") we use it as a learning opportunity, especially in terms of tying any required behavior change to our client's priorities and commitments.

Reflecting back on what we've already identified as the most crucial aspects of psychotherapeutic success—namely seeing through the client's worldview, dynamic dialogical responsiveness, a collaborative/egalitarian relationship, freedom from normative judgment (unconditional acceptance), and therapist authenticity—it becomes readily apparent that when we *embody* the policies, values, and practices of an institution we all but sacrifice these perspectives and practices so crucial to such a therapeutic alliance. Even if one has some degree of "insight" into the problem that an institutional lens is in the therapeutic relationship (which is a big "if"), the illusion is that one can turn off his/her institutional and professional agency when entering into the psychotherapeutic arena with the client. Thus institutionalized, we see our clients through this lens; the way our client appears is an obvious truth, reality, or "is"—as if we're seeing our client as they really "are"—rather than a "showing up" (appearance). One thing that the postmodernists had in common with the Communist thinkers was in the recognition that our consciousness—including the contents of our mind and the perceptions that we experience—is a product of the social arenas in which we participate. Karl Marx (1904) wrote:

> It is not the consciousness of men that determines their being, but, on the contrary, their social being determines their consciousness. (11–12)

So yes, reality is socially constructed; but, not randomly. It's clear that powerful interests have adapted to democracy by shaping public opinion. Edward Bernays, Sigmund Freud's nephew, also known as the father of public relations, believed that the unconscious was indeed running the show and that the public needed to hear the right messages—largely in the form of advertising. Whether by government or corporation, public opinion had to be under control of the "enlightened" few. Corporate heads ("manufacturing need" by way of marketing/advertising), Woodrow Wilson (mobilizing public support for World War I), and Joseph Goebbels (Nazi minister of anti-Semitic propaganda) utilized Bernays's methods of shaping the public's opinion and behavior by manipulating images and emotions. The rest is history.

I say all this to emphasize how our minds are a product of our conversations and with all good intentions we can lose all perspective simply by participating in institutional rhetoric—and be totally unaware of this process.

Of course we can't run an institution without an institutional vocabulary. But in recognizing the phenomenon of institutionalization we can see to it that the institutional vocabulary and practices should not enter into the therapeutic relationship with the client. This is tricky. We need to insist on the separation between the sacred (human-to-human intimate contact) and the profane (administration). There needs to be existential space protected within and from the institutional framework. Much the way tech companies create playful environments for their creative people to create.

We'll now turn our attention to how professional specialization vis-à-vis specialized vocabularies became means of asserting power, dominating others, and social control.

MICHEL FOUCAULT—KNOWLEDGE AND NIETZSCHE'S WILL TO POWER

Another aspect of our reality that is transparent to us (i.e., we cannot see it) is the way in which the Enlightenment rationalist and scientific worldviews have structured our lives. One of the ways we impose a rational ordering of the world is to classify and categorize. This practice is automatic, yet we're hardly aware what it means or its consequences; and moreover we view their products as truth itself, i.e., we view the abstractions as having an existence independent of the particularities from which they've arisen. Stars and galaxies (concrete particularities) exist, but constellations (abstractions) don't exist the way stars and galaxies exist. Constellations are abstractions that appear to have an independent physical existence, when in fact, their "existence" is wholly dependent on a particular point of view (e.g., from earth) and a label (e.g., Orion). So go psychiatric diagnoses!

This is a form of metaphysics—a product of the phenomenon of reification—that has heretofore been little scrutinized. The speaking of an abstraction such as "schizophrenia" is to posit a metaphysical (i.e., non-material) entity inside a person, reify an abstract term into a "thing" with the ability to cause observable "symptoms," totalize the person as a schizophrenic (or "having" schizophrenia), and marginalize the person and minimize everything else that's important about that person. This is true despite (1) how experts have been unable to point to physical neural causes/correlates or genetic markers and (2) the fields of complexity neuroscience and epigenetics (i.e., the study of how our thinking, feeling, behaving, lifestyle, and environment alter the expression of our DNA; chapter 9) have established that genetics and childhood conditioning are propensity not destiny. But underneath this putative search for knowledge there is something else going on with this labeling.

Michel Foucault (1983), a disciple of Friedrich Nietzsche, observed that the relationship between expert and non-expert has to do with power and submission, respectively. This is true in terms of the "expert" possessing exclusive knowledge in comparison with the non-expert and in terms of the "expert" defining the "non-expert." The imposition of expert knowledge *on* "the other," or more specifically the act of classifying, is a pecking-into-order. When a person is labeled either "mentally ill" (or any of its diagnoses) or "criminal" the existential effect is to elevate the expert and marginalize the non-expert (the person to whom the label is applied).

As if the imposition of psychiatric labels wasn't bad enough given their self-fulfilling consequences, it is also a marginalization of the person's experience. Far from an egalitarian relationship, the transaction is characteristically subjugating. The client is demanded upon to passively accept the pathological label and with it the normative worldview, all of which is implicit in the label. Furthermore, labels by their very nature are totalizing; they act as a lens from which everything a person does is interpreted. These labels, internalized and identified with, appear as a totalizing reality for the person who has now been transformed into a "patient." For Foucault power is internalized in this way, and as such, by simply using the professional vocabulary (e.g., "I have bipolar disorder.") we unknowingly participate in our own subjugation (i.e., forced submission to control by others) and marginalization (i.e., relegation to a lower social standing).

Thus we arrive at Nietzsche's will to power. According to Nietzsche, underneath the thin film of niceties, formalities, manners, "rationality," professional roles, and stability of civilization in general is a seething cauldron of clashing wills. The expert—like all other cultural agents—is compelled to impose her/his expertise on the non-expert. The non-expert has no choice but to submit or rebel. This is simply a phenomenon of enculturation. The values and ways of living considered "normal" or "healthy" (i.e., those of the therapist/psychiatrist)—often reflecting the manipulation of those in power—are imposed on the other (the client). According to Harlene Anderson (1997):

> The dominant voice, the culturally designated professional voice, usually speaks and decides for marginal populations—gender, economic, ethnic, religious, political, and racial minorities—whether therapy is indicated and, if so, which therapy and toward what purpose. Sometimes unwittingly, sometimes knowingly, therapists subjugate or sacrifice a client to the influences of this broader context, which is primarily patriarchal, authoritarian, and hierarchical. (71)

As mental health professionals are unwitting agents of both cultural and professional discourse this is sometimes interpreted by philosophers (e.g., Foucault and Thomas Szasz) as social control involving punishment (albeit insidious and indirect) of the deviant. Again, not to be too hard on mental health professionals, this clashing of wills happens in all relationships. However, in the mental health profession the imposition of cultural norms, morality, and values are hidden beneath the guise of scientific neutrality and objectivity, which includes often colloquially judging behavior as to its "appropriateness." Gary Gutting (2013) writing in the *Stanford Encyclopedia of Philosophy*, said:

> But, according to Foucault, the new idea that the mad were merely sick ("mentally" ill) and in need of medical treatment was not at all a clear improvement on earlier conceptions (e.g., the Renaissance idea that the mad were in contact with the mysterious forces of cosmic tragedy or the seventeenth–eighteenth-century view of madness as a renouncing of reason). Moreover, he argued that the alleged scientific neutrality of modern medical treatments of insanity in fact covers for controlling challenges to a conventional bourgeois morality. In short, Foucault argued that what was presented as an objective, incontrovertible scientific discovery (that madness is mental illness) was in fact the product of eminently questionable social and ethical commitments.

Foucault saw people as different and that these differences should be embraced. Both Foucault and Szasz recognized the fundamental equality between all human beings and the need to relate to people as equals, adult to adult, subject to subject.

As we will see in the next chapter on the work of Korteling (2014)—which should be all but self-evident from experience—when we label brain processes that involve thought, feeling, perception, judgment, etc., we're really labeling identities. Saying a person "has bipolar disorder" is not the same as saying someone has an ulcer. Understood rightly, the psychiatric medicalization of persons' identities and the resulting marginalization constitutes *social injustice*. Like other non-dominant groups, consumers of mental health services are in a place to resist their subjugation in favor of equality and social justice. Moreover, this is not merely a case of being politically correct and using the right words (though it does involve this); the entire context must be promulgated in order for the truth of our common lot and fundamental equality—from the point of view of human subjectivity—to be recognized.

The postmodernists, while recognizing the fundamental equality of persons, view people and their identities as embodiments of competing social discourses. We're embodied instances of culture looking to prevail and thus replicate themselves. Despite references to reason or consensus, what do you think is happening when couples fight over whether or not the lights in rooms that are not being used should be turned off or not? This imposition of our judgments, values, and ways of living may be good for parenting children, but not negotiating relationships or for empowering adults. As Susan Blackmore (1999) puts it, we're meme machines. Memes are defined as the basic units of culture. Or as John Gaventa (2003) adds, "Power constitutes agents rather than being deployed by them" (3). In other words, our own private spontaneous thoughts or spoken expressions reflect that which has been imprinted on us. This is easier to see in our judgments of others. In other words, in our judgments of "the other" we perpetuate our own subjugation—which was imposed on us early on—despite it "seeming like" an expression of our own self-authorship or free will.

The same is true in our own self-descriptions. When we think or say, "I have a mental illness" or "I'm an ex-con" we participate in our own subjugation and marginalization. For an excellent and accessible description of memes and memetics I recommend Richard Brodie's (the original creator of Microsoft Word) *Viruses of the Mind* (1996).

As we have seen in chapter 5 every word in a vocabulary communicates its context, and in light of Foucault and Nietzsche, its context of power relations and subjugating practices. Never before the postmodern language paradigm has the power of a single word been recognized.

The pathologizing vocabulary of "expert knowledge" affects the helping relationship in another way. The professional, or persons in general, experiences the will to power in what they notice about the client (or the other). When a therapist is captured by the normative lens what s/he *sees* in addition to "symptoms" when they see their clients is deficiencies: co-dependency, incompetence, fragility, chemical dependency, controlling, inability to assert oneself, inability to regulate one's emotions, etc. The social control or dominating discourse stance is to move this deviation to normality—personally experienced by the therapist/psychiatrist (being unwitting agents of normative culture themselves) as a subtle or not-so-subtle judgment and disdain toward the client or the client's behavior along with the necessity for "treatment" or, in some general sense, reformation. This is in contrast to the postmodern non-normative relational stance which is similar to Carl Rogers's unconditional positive regard—a very expansive point of view of loving and accepting people exactly as they are. Dissatisfaction with the way people are comes from a different point of view.

In a collaborative and artful helping relationship we work within the client's frame of reference to discover where they're interested and motivated already (versus "motivational enhancement" toward "normality") and then find ways in which they are already moving in that direction, all the while looking for and building on very small change in the client's preferred direction (giving plenty of room for ambivalence along the way). Recall that complexity neuroscience has definitively concluded that neural change is *incremental*. Blinded to incremental change—by deficit-based categories—you can't build on incremental change.

Moreover getting outside the normative Western discourse we see other peoples, other cultures, now or in times past, "advanced" or "primitive" all as making full use of the brain's ability to adapt to its environment. Whether we're talking about people who break the law to get what they want (aka criminals), ancient Samarians, third world countries, etc., if we look close enough we see the complexity of the brain creating practical distinctions in language. Insoo Kim Berg (personal communication, June 1999), an originator of solution-focused therapy, used to say that a single mother living in poverty in a disadvantaged area solves hundreds of problems a day. The perfection and grandeur of the human condition in all its various manifestations is concealed by the normalizing discourses, most notably, ironically, and unfortunately those of mental health.

A deficit-based clinical worldview is founded on a normative framework, not on a client's strengths. The world of neuroplasticity starts with client strengths and works, through repetitive practice, along with an appreciation for incremental progress, project upon project, toward the accomplishment of desired objectives. Additionally, it should be clear that eliciting and amplifying what the client is already doing that's working in terms of getting what they want (i.e., eliciting and amplifying exceptions) is a big boost to self-confidence. By being a weapon of normative discourse the mental health profession has been complicit with the dominant cultural discourse's maintenance of power relations and manufacturing of discontent.

In summary, the Enlightenment project of analysis and categorization (read: objectification of persons) was not only an attempt at understanding but also a power play. Knowing that our sublimated instinct for domination is at play in our purported attempts to help people would at least give us some choice in the matter and an opportunity to orient ourselves toward a collaborative and egalitarian relationship. This kind of subject-to-subject relationship recognizes our common subjective dilemma, how we're all in the same boat.

Divesting the Diagnostic and Statistical Manual (DSM) of its truth status, we can see more clearly how the psychiatric vocabulary defines and marginalizes people as well as asserting role and power relations between them. Yet even without the advantage of this point of view, as we will see in the next chapter, the very makers of the DSM have come to see its fatal flaws.

LABELING IS LETHAL TO RELATIONSHIPS

Again, as the clinical world is a self-enclosed, self-affirming reality with all its taken-for-granted truths it is unable to look critically at the consequences of its vocabulary and practices. Or additionally or alternatively, because the clinical world is viewed as objectively true (due to reification and an unwarranted link to scientific legitimacy) we might think these effects, though unfortunate, inevitable. For example, the mental health profession creates its stigmas then tries to mitigate their damage. No distinction of "mentally ill," no stigma. We all suffer from the human condition and anyone not trapped in the clinical reality of mental health and with an ounce of humility and perspective would see this.

Another area where "diagnostic" labels are particularly damaging is in personal and professional relationships. A crucial aspect of relationships is that they involve the reconciliation of differing points of view. Moreover, as I mention throughout this book, by and large, human beings in the early twenty-first century are simply instruments of culture, instances of culture looking to impose itself and replicate itself—i.e., their values, ways of living, etc.—in other people. What do you think the *judgmental mind,* with all its certainty, is all about? The Nietzschean will to power and ensuing clash of wills is inevitable. This often is described in relationships as "having to be right."

However, when one partner in a relationship has a known mental health history with a "diagnosis," the other person's will to power is only too happy to seize advantage of this built-in, ready-to-hand marginalization. The person with the "diagnosis" has a credibility problem right from the get-go in the battle of "who's right." Furthermore, as was mentioned in the section above ("Foucault"), psychiatric diagnoses enjoy the cover of scientific neutrality while they—in reality, as normative conceptions—serve as the dominant culture's critique of unconventionality. Psychiatric diagnoses are the "nuclear option" in relationship conflict.

This naturally feeds into the very common human phenomenon that when in the heat of an argument we see the other person's viewpoint as absurd, irrational, or in various ways distorted. In a world where the recognition of subjectivity is the purview of so few, expansive empathy is in short supply. When conflict ensues often we see the other person as unreasonable or irrational in their perspective and resulting action. A psychiatric diagnosis is a very efficient catalyst to this process of invalidating the other's point of view in a very permanent way. Furthermore, family and friends, forever with the paranoid radar set to detect "symptoms" and "relapses" (where they are and where they aren't), are quick in the face of the all-too-human slothfulness, anger, sluggishness, staying up all night, excitability, avoidance, worrisomeness, irritability, etc., with the quip: "Have you been taking your medications?" We live in a "chemical imbalance"/medication-centered universe.

Herein lies the "crazy making" that goes on in relationships, families, and notably in the mental health profession. The very understandable upsets, fears, frustrations, and sensitivities of life and relationships—even if highly exaggerated by the heat of emotion—are labeled as symptoms of a "mental illness." Once this happens the so-called "normal" person involved stops listening and stops taking the person with the so-called "psychiatric diagnosis" seriously. We all know what it is like when we're not taken seriously or our point of view is invalidated—we go through the roof! This is one of the ways I've noted that "mental illness" is constructed and maintained socially. People under the influence of the clinical world and diagnoses literally, in a self-fulfilling way, create the very "symptoms" they don't like (in the case of families or friends) or are purportedly there to help with (in the case of mental health professionals). A person struggling to be heard and taken seriously among a sea of professionals who can only see through the "diagnostic" label is like Kevin McCarthy in the 1956 classic *Invasion of the Body Snatchers*.

In our vocabularically realized institutionalization we lose our humanity. Again, not to be too hard on the mental health profession, this zombie-like (to use a Heideggerian term) institutionalized state is everywhere, in all institutions and cultures. The "criminal justice" system with its totalizing labels (criminal, ex-con, felon, etc.) is similarly oblivious to the effects of its language. It is the state of humanity. Yet, the mental health or coaching professions should be at the vanguard of doing something about this state of affairs.

When it comes to relationships, the label is like a straightjacket that one is never free of. The people in our lives "see" and are forever on the lookout for the behaviors that confirm the label and then respond accordingly. A very self-conscious (in the case of the person-client) and other-conscious (in the case of significant others and mental health professionals) *paranoia* sets in as the "symptom/relapse" radar is forever on high alert. Recall that you get more of what you focus on. Even when these behaviors are not present, it's seen as the "diagnosis in remission" or brief "flights into health" or "in recovery"—all of which presuppose an invisible condition that could threaten a comeback at any time.

It's like putting a curse on someone. Perhaps in the beginning, unsure of the veracity of curses, the cursed person begins to interpret everyday random "bad happenings" to be signs of the truth of the curse. This curse focus itself (like a diagnosis focus) throws people off their game, thus making it more likely that they will be more vulnerable to making mistakes from the start. As more mistakes happen they are readily seen as confirming the reality of the curse, which makes the person even more anxious, thus more likely to make more mistakes, and, in turn, further confirming the "curse." If there is one thing to be definitively said about psychiatric diagnoses, it is that they are self-fulfilling—this is what they have in common with curses.

This is how primitive we really still are. The well-intentioned priests with their symbols of legitimacy (PhDs, MDs, LCSWs) along with the pretense of scientific authority, social sanction (legitimacy bestowed by society by virtue of being a profession), and with sufficient gravitas (an invention of ancient Rome) declare things, true or not, and these things that they declare carry great weight, especially with the vulnerable individual. A weight that one can carry his or her entire life (see chapter 9, "The Creation of the Patient").

Trapped in a sea of ready-to-hand labels (co-dependent, bipolar, controlling, lazy, manipulative, schizophrenic, alcoholic, borderline personality disorder, bully, addict, antisocial personality, racist, etc.) that are self-/other-defeating and self-fulfilling we are—professional and non-professional alike—*developmentally arrested* in terms of the perspectives and skillsets needed to hold others accountable (when appropriate), to reconcile differences, to encourage *interdependence,* to inspire, to support harmony in a relationship, to jointly run a household, to jointly parent, and to, in general, nurture a relationship. The use of labels effectively takes its user "off the hook" and off the playing field of intersubjectivity the very domain of our ability to respectfully influence one another. The label is like some kind of club that we use to incite people into "treatment" or into some kind of reformation. With the use of labels—*spoken or not spoken,* it doesn't matter when they're integrated into your perceptions—power is permanently vested in the so-called "normal" person, ironically to their own detriment and the detriment of the relationship.

NOTE

1. *The Hollow Men* by T. S. Elliot (1925).

SEVEN

The DSM Criticized by Its Makers (Applies Equally to ICD)

The advent of the Diagnostic Statistical Manual, fifth edition (DSM-5; May 2013) is nothing less than an act of hubris and greed on the part of the pharmaceutical industry. As is declared in Proverbs 16:18, "Pride goeth before destruction, and an haughty spirit before a fall." Like any other act of hubris its overreaching reveals what it has been doing all along. The audacity of the creators of the DSM-5 to pathologize an ever-broader range of human behavior—especially in children—has brought critics out of the woodwork, non-professional and professional alike, in particular and notably are the creators of the DSM.

Allen Frances, MD, chair of the DSM-IV Task Force and author of *Saving Normal: An Insider's Revolt against Out-of-Control Psychiatric Diagnosis, DSM-5, Big Pharma, and the Medicalization of Ordinary Life,* has led the charge against the excesses of the DSM-5 and DSM in general. From his own experience supervising the development of the DSM-IV, Frances (2010) learned firsthand the dangers of *diagnostic inflation*:

> Our panel tried hard to be conservative and careful but inadvertently contributed to three false "epidemics"—attention deficit disorder, autism and childhood bipolar disorder. Clearly, our net was cast too wide and captured many "patients" who might have been far better off never entering the mental health system.

Astute and discerning professionals, Frances among them, could see that the boundaries between "normal" and "abnormal" were indeed "fuzzy" and more than likely were artificial markers imposed on a normal-abnormal continuum. The current crisis of *diagnostic hyperinflation* in the DSM-5—a reflection of the arbitrary nature of the DSM's categorical boundaries—had its roots early in the DSM's development:

> Psychiatric diagnosis is facing a renewed crisis of confidence caused by diagnostic inflation. The boundaries of psychiatry are easily expanded because no bright line separates patients who are simply worried from those with mild mental disorders. The DSM-III opened the door to loose diagnosis by defining conditions that were no more than slightly more severe versions of such everyday problems as mild depression, generalized anxiety, social anxiety, simple phobias, sexual dysfunctions, and sleep disorders. (Frances, 2013b, 221)

Frances was astounded by the unrestrained loosening of criteria for current diagnoses and the invention of new ones in the DSM-5, all of which would undoubtedly result in the pathologizing and unnecessary medicating of tens of millions of normal people. Changes incorporated into the DSM-5 included one eating binge per month qualifying as "binge eating disorder," expansive loosening of the criteria for adult attention deficit/hyperactivity disorder, normal grief = major depressive disorder, normal age-related forgetfulness = mild neurocognitive disorder, strange thinking = psychosis risk syndrome, normal worry about medical illness = somatic symptom disorder, the normal frustrations of everyday life = mixed anxiety depression, normal eccentricities in children = autistic spectrum disorder, etc. (Frances, 2013b). Understanding the humanitarian risk and consequences of such changes Frances (2013a) realized his moral obligation to "Save Normal":

> It was not just a matter of DSM-V having a closed and secretive process; it would likely produce a very dangerous product. . . . DSM-V was going to create public health problems, and the public needed to have a say. . . . DSM-V was too important to be left in the hands of a group of well-meaning, but badly misguided, "experts." (loc. 157)

Allen Frances was an insider in another way; he was a "thought leader" for over two decades for the pharmaceutical industry. In the pharmaceutical industry "thought leaders" allegedly "educate" professionals about the benefits of their drugs. Spending twice as much money on promotion than research, drug company symposia and in-service trainings are pretexts for aggressive marketing of drugs developed by research of the "wrong kind . . . done in the wrong way, and with the wrong motives—avoiding lines of inquiry that might actually teach us something important" (Frances 2013a, 89).

All this begs the question of how or if the American Psychiatric Association (APA) was influenced by big pharma in their DSM-5 diagnostic decisions; or even if economic interest and/or simple shortsightedness resulted in such reckless behavior. Though Frances (2013a) doesn't definitively answer these questions, he certainly alludes to how the pharmaceutical industry has shaped the minds of the psychiatric profession:

> In recent decades, the drug companies have efficiently hijacked the medical enterprise by exerting undue influence on the decisions made

> by doctors, patients, scientists, journals, professional associations, consumer advocacy groups, pharmacists, insurance companies, politicians, bureaucrats, and administrators. And the best way to sell psychotropic pills is to sell psychiatric ills. . . . Many doctors are witting or unwitting agents in the pervasive drug company marketing campaign to sell new diagnoses. "Education" and "research" can become sheep's clothing covering what is really a wolfish marketing pitch. A large stable of psychiatry's "thought leaders" are recruited to help drumbeat the wondrous benefits that accrue from drugs and to downplay the harms. . . . Pharma used thought leaders to exert dominance over psychiatry and research programs. The dozens of industry-sponsored symposia at the annual meeting of the American Psychiatric Association offered the best speakers and the only food and attracted the biggest audiences. Most of weekly grand rounds held at hospitals and medical schools throughout the country were funded by Pharma and led by big-name faculty conveniently supplied by its "speakers' bureaus." (91–92)

Worse still many of the authors of the DSM have had financial ties to the pharmaceutical industry. Robert Whitaker and Lisa Cosgrove (2015) summarize Cosgrove's (2006) article titled, "Financial Ties between DSM-IV Panel Members and the Pharmaceutical Industry":

> Many of the authors of the DSM manuals, as they drew up these diagnostic boundaries, had financial ties to the industry, serving on advisory boards and as consultants to the pharmaceutical companies that made the products that would be sold to these diagnostic groups. At least 56 percent of the DSM-IV panel members had financial ties to a drug company, and this conflict of interest was particularly pronounced on panels for psychiatric conditions where a medication was recommended as a first-line therapy. One hundred percent of the DSM-IV panels for "mood disorders" and for "schizophrenia and other psychotic disorders" had a conflict. Eighty-one percent of the "anxiety disorders" panel did, and 62 percent of the panel for "disorders usually first diagnosed in infancy, childhood or adolescence." (loc. 2018)

The issue of the intentions and motivations of the APA creators of the DSM-5 aside, their diagnostic decisions certainly played into the hands of big pharma. Having been intimately associated with both sides, Frances (2013b) was in a unique position to elucidate their unholy alliance:

> Drug companies take marketing advantage of the loose DSM definitions by promoting the misleading idea that everyday life problems are actually undiagnosed psychiatric illnesses caused by a chemical imbalance and require a solution in pill form. (221)

Note that Frances's critique of the DSM is especially poignant because he was the lead designer of the DSM-IV. He deplores the real-world human consequences and corrupt motives for the expansion of the diagnostic criteria. However, we will see that the meaninglessness, arbitrariness, and destructive consequences of the DSM go far beyond what Allen Frances has imagined.

Now let's turn our attention to the DSM's reliability and validity, variables without which the DSM is meaningless. Reliability means how reliably do different raters using the same written criteria come up with the same "diagnosis" when viewing the same person. Validity means how accurately do the psychiatric definitions reflect the constructs they are purported to describe.

Carol Tavris in her 2013 *Wall Street Journal* article describes how Gary Greenberg, psychotherapist, field researcher for the DSM, and author of *Manufacturing Depression*, was appalled by the DSM-5's lack of reliability:

> And he [Greenberg] was there when those scientific aspirations met reality and all hell broke loose. Mr. Greenberg gives us a front-row seat at the APA's annual meeting in 2011, when results of the field trials were reported. Field trials are intended to test the reliability of diagnostic criteria—meaning that two psychiatrists observing the same person's symptoms should have a pretty good chance of agreeing on a diagnosis. But the results were dismal. Agreement on identifying even Major Depressive Disorder and Generalized Anxiety Disorder—what Mr. Greenberg calls the "Dodge Dart and Ford Falcon of the DSM, simple and reliable and ubiquitous" disorders—was low. Moreover, the field testing on patients failed miserably: 5,000 clinicians signed up to participate, 195 finished training for it, and only 70 enrolled any patients in trials. The APA tried to put a good spin on these numbers—"nearly 150 patients have joined the study"—ignoring, Mr. Greenberg notes, that their goal was 10,000. Only two months before the data had to be in, the clinician field trials had barely begun.

Frances (2013b) chimed in:

> I found the DSM-5 process secretive, closed, and disorganized. Deadlines were consistently missed. Field trials produced reliability results that did not meet historical standards. . . . The APA refused a petition for an independent scientific review of the DSM-5 that was endorsed by more than fifty mental health associations (9). Publishing profits trumped public interest. (221)

Moreover the evidence is overwhelming that there is a continuum between what's considered "normal" and what's considered "pathological." Thus, DSM categories are artificial; the lines drawn between normal and abnormal are completely arbitrary and very "fuzzy."

Low reliability though certainly a problem is nothing compared to the DSM's all-out failure in terms of validity. The "diagnoses" are not valid concepts in that they are meaningless, they tell us nothing about the nature of the problem or its solution. In the lead up to the DSM-5, Steven Hyman, member of the DSM-5 Task Force and chair of the International

Advisory Group on the Revision of ICD-10 (International Statistical Classification of Diseases, 10th ed.), admits:

> Overall, there is evidence that the current diagnoses and their corresponding sets of criteria fall short of mapping nature. . . . Owing to the limited understanding of the biological underpinnings of mental disorders that neuroscience and genetics could provide at the time, the diagnoses within the DSM-III and the DSM-IV have necessarily been based on clinical observation. Despite the optimism of Robins and Guze, laboratory tests for the major, common psychiatric disorders have not yet materialized. (2007, 727)

Or, if we consult Allen Frances (2013a), the chairperson of the DSM-IV:

> The expectation that there would be a simple gene or neurotransmitter or circuitry explanation for any mental disorder has turned out to be naïve and illusory. (10)

Nassir Ghaemi, MD, Tufts Medical School Department of Psychiatry, in his "Requiem for DSM" in the *Psychiatric Times* (2013) put it eloquently:

> When I graduated a generation ago, I accepted DSM IV as if it were the truth. I trusted that my elders would put the truth first, and then compromise for practical purposes where they had no truths to follow. It took me two decades to realize a painful truth, spoke now frankly by those who gave us the DSM III when Ronald Reagan was elected, and by those who gave us DSM IV when Bill Clinton was president: the leaders of those DSMs don't believe there are scientific truths in psychiatric diagnoses—only mutually agreed upon falsehoods. They call it reliability.

Put simply, by the admission of its authors, the DSM diagnoses are simply labels attached to sets of behaviors (symptoms) with absolutely no reference to a causal disease, the very construct the diagnoses purport to represent. In other words, unlike other medical conditions, the psychiatric diagnostic categories represent "symptoms" without a known "disease"! However, the conventional wisdom in response to this criticism is that we just haven't found the cause and we need better tools; this constitutes the "precision medicine" movement. But to think this way in terms of one-way causality, that all that is happening is that some area of the brain is causing the "symptoms," is to be completely oblivious of the reality of neuroplasticity.

To say that in some general way the mind/brain is the cause of emotions, thinking, and behavior is only half of the picture—the picture that the "doctor" and "patient," embedded in the clinical reality, see as the whole picture. It would be better said that there are always neural *correlates* to emotions, thinking, and behavior. Importantly, as is demonstrated throughout this book, the converse is also true, that different language, thinking, and behavior alter the mind/brain. The difference between *causation* and *correlation* is the difference between the metaphors of "chemical imbalance" and "neuroplasticity," respectively, both of which represent entirely different realities and possibilities. Correlation in this case means dual causality or reflexivity. In other words, the "wild goose chase" of "precision medicine" to "map nature," to find the exact neuronal or genetic cause of various "disorders," is a complete waste of time.

Furthermore, the old "nature versus nurture" controversy when it comes to human behavior is no longer valid in light of epigenetics and neuroplasticity. When the rest of us discover the power of language we'll stop parsing infinitesimally and obsessively the minutia of the genetics and biochemistry of the brain (which is the main thrust of "precision medicine"). It was evolution that gave us the DNA—which itself is changeable in its expression—that gave us this amazingly malleable brain; stop analyzing the hardware and get on with mastering the software, which is the direct source of the power of the human brain!

On the other hand, if "precision medicine" can *seriously* include contextual variables, like environment and lifestyle (as it purports to do), they may come around to complexity neuroscience, neuroplasticity, and epigenetics. But I wouldn't hold my breath as like other holistic movements (e.g., recovery, wellness) they get superficially layered over the rock-hard realities of the clinical and diagnostic world.

Let's take a close look at the logic of psychiatric diagnoses and in the process enter the Twilight Zone. If you operationally define the causal entity (disease or diagnosis) in terms of the effects (symptoms) and you can't identify a physical cause "in nature" then what you're left with is a logical fallacy of circular reasoning. In effect, since the "disease" is defined solely by its "symptoms" (a more-or-less characteristic cluster of behaviors and subjective experiences), then the "symptoms" (as sole definition of the "diagnosis") are causing the "symptoms" and "up is down, and down is up" and "we're all mad here" (two apropos references from Lewis Carroll's *Alice in Wonderland*, 2009)!

However, the nature of language, grammar, communication, and the human mind don't allow us to see this, and what happens instead is through the routine use of these words in conversations ("We're looking for an effective treatment for schizophrenia." "He's taking medications for his depression.") the mind manufactures in its constitutive imagination a "thing," a metaphysical non-substance that we keep going after with the shotgun approach of pharmaceuticals. This is called reification, to make into a reality. This is why we can be so sure of the presence of an identifiable, measurable, and consistent biological substrate or disease—implied in the sentences used—causing the symptoms even though there isn't one. Martin Heidegger (1959/1971), probably the most influential philosopher of the twentieth century and one of the progenitors of the "linguistic turn" in philosophy, asserted:

> Words, like the chisel of the carver, can create what never existed before rather than simply describe what already exists. As a man speaks, not only is the thing which he is declaring coming into existence, but also the man himself.

In other words, in the repetitive uttering of "psychiatric diagnoses" not only is the "diagnosis" made into a reality, so are the complementary "professional" (aka expert) and "the patient" identities.

In his more recent article, "The Diagnosis of Mental Disorders: The Problem of Reification," Hyman (2010) in his introduction uses the following epigram:

> The tendency has always been strong to believe that whatever received a name must be an entity or being, having an independent existence of its own.
>
> —John Stuart Mill (156)

This is a fact that professionals have at best forgotten, or at worst were never made clearly aware of. Whereas the public was *never* made aware of this. Call it mass denial or mass delusion. Recall, the ancient Greeks did the same thing with their gods, including attributing them as causes of irrational behavior. Clearly a man before his time, Thomas Szasz (1970/1991) saw this clearly, albeit without the postmodern perspective:

> Instead of calling attention to conflicting human needs, aspirations, and values, the concept of mental illness provides an amoral and impersonal "thing"—an "Illness"—as an explanation for problems in living. We may recall in this connection that not so long ago it was devils and witches that were held responsible for man's problems in living. The belief in mental illness, as something other than man's trouble in getting along with his fellow man, is the proper heir to the belief in witchcraft. Mental illness thus exists or is "real" in exactly the same sense in which witchcraft existed or was "real." (21)

The gods, witches, devils, mental illness, and human superstitions or prejudices in general were/are made real simply through constant and customary reference to them and their narrative context in speaking.

The way language, grammar, and subjectivity work when we say, "She has schizophrenia" or "He is struggling with bipolar disorder" or "The standard of care for the treatment of depression is" or "People can recover from mental illness" we are bringing a non-material, non-existing entity into existence and all those concerned act accordingly. The sentences presuppose the reality of the label; by speaking and responding to these sentences (and thousands of similar ones) we "rubberstamp" the presuppositions embedded in them. This reification is key in creating the patient identity, in the words of Korteling (2014):

> One way in which DSM-labels affect people lies in the way people interpret these labels. People tend to interpret DSM labels as things that

> exist (reification), and this interpretation interferes with one's social and self-constructed identity, whereby the "mentally ill"–label eventually defines these identities (Grover, 2005). (89)

No one is disputing that all feeling, thinking, and behavior has neural correlates. The truth is that the human brain is a complex system whose main emergent property is that of language and interpretation. With the right language and practice the brain is capable of better addressing itself (in its lower manifestations) and its outside circumstances. This amazing process is short-circuited by the manufacture and maintenance of a mythological and causal "disease."

The little bit of benefit—albeit far outweighed by the cost—of the DSM labels is known as *heuristic* or practical benefit. In other words, certain psychotherapeutic techniques or psychiatric medications target certain "symptoms"; the "diagnosis" is shorthand for the symptoms, ergo the "diagnosis" is useful. In the words of Hyman himself:

> The disorders contained therein are heuristics that have proven extremely useful in clinical practice and research, especially by creating a common language. . . . Unfortunately, the disorders within these classifications are not generally treated as heuristic, but to a great degree have become reified. Disorders within the DSM-IV or ICD-10 are often treated as if they were natural kinds, real entities that exist independently of any particular rater (Kendell & Jablensky 2003). (2010, 156)

Of course, you could get the heuristic value by just using a few representative behaviors ("symptoms"), thereby avoiding reifying the label; but absent the postmodern perspective the power of language is all but hidden. Furthermore, as we will discover in the chapter on postmodern coaching, *you get more of what you focus on*; thus focusing on undesirable behaviors and experiences while trying to help someone can't help but bring more of that unwanted behavior and subjective experience. Recall just using the pathologizing labels—spoken aloud to others or silently to oneself—is sufficient focus to manifest this creation. Moreover, when we focus on what people *want*—i.e., *not* on what they don't want—we tap into the power of human intentionality, commitment, passion, vision, and agency.

Paula Caplan (another professional contributor to the DSM) in her book *So They Say You're Crazy* (1995) asserts that such labeling is at best irrelevant to helping someone feel and perform better in life.

> The professionals most concerned with labeling claim that they assign people to categories of mental illness so that they will know how to help them. If such assignments to categories really did help very much, that would indeed be encouraging, but treatment of emotional problems and conflicts is very different from medical or surgical treatment. If I broke a limb, I would want to be properly diagnosed as having a broken arm so that the surgeon would not mistakenly set and put a cast

> on my leg. But diagnosing individuals as mentally ill has not been shown to do much to alleviate their anguish and indeed often makes it worse. (12)

To reiterate, psychiatric diagnoses disable people by misleading them (and the professionals) into thinking that the nature of the problem is some "diagnosis" and/or "chemical imbalance" (conveniently for the pharmaceutical industry) as the cause of their disturbing emotions and counterproductive behaviors. As it turns out the chosen *metaphor* for understanding behavior and emotional difficulties is the single most important element in helping people change. So it is critical that we find the right one. Moreover, the power of metaphors, and the power of language more generally, is that they construct reality.

Allen Frances (2013a) admits psychiatric diagnoses are constructs (not "myths," a common misinterpretation of Thomas Szasz) and that we need constructs:

> Mental constructs of reality are imperfect, but indispensable, ways to organize the otherwise bewildering phenomena of the world. . . . Mental disorders are not real diseases . . . but neither are they dangerous myths . . . we are constantly constructing perceptions and finding temporary meanings that are useful, but never completely accurate. . . . Schizophrenia is a useful construct—not myth, not disease. It is a description of a particular set of psychiatric problems, *not an explanation of their cause*. . . . It is good to know and use the DSM definitions, but not to reify or worship them. (21; my italics added)

If psychiatric diagnoses are "not an explanation of their cause" (Frances, DSM-IV chairman) and they "don't map nature" (Hyman, DSM-5 Task Force member and chair of the International Advisory Group on the Revision of ICD-10) why on earth are they called "diagnoses"? They tell us nothing and they influence everything. This now is the consensus, but the DSM still maintains its authority! Reason has gone completely out the window!

So here is where Allen Frances and I part ways. No one is denying that people have emotional and cognitive problems leading to difficulty living and vice versa, not even Thomas Szasz. Nor are we denying the intransigence of these difficulties (which can better be explained by complexity neuroscience). Frances is still stuck in the medical paradigm and therefore can't see beyond the reductionist need to label something as broken or abnormal. In the postmodern worldview we are free from such deficit-based language and thus unfettered we use a human language of empowerment and wisdom to realize the lives we desire. Frances is a prime example of how in its early stages of comprehension and realization, the postmodern framework lives as a chimera (any mythical animal with parts taken from various animals, from *New Oxford English Dictionary*, 2001) pasted together with modernist constructions of truth.

The National Institute of Mental Health response to the DSM debacle and its "fuzzy" categories has been the aforementioned attempt at "precision medicine." They admit symptoms and DSM diagnoses imply only superficial similarities: a dolphin is not a fish. According to the logic of precision medicine, categories are useful to the extent that they infer a cause and therefore treatment. So let's dig deeper with more sophisticated technology into genetic markers or expand more broadly into sociocultural causes. Steven Pinker (1997) describes the difference between "fuzzy" and "crisp" categories:

> Fuzzy [artificial] categories come from examining objects and unsightfully recording the correlations among their features. Their predictive power comes from similarity: if A shares some features with B, it probably shares others. They work by recording the clusters in reality. Well-defined categories [natural or "crisp"], in contrast, work by ferreting out theories that capture people's best guess about what makes the world tick. Their predictive power comes from deduction: if A implies [causes] B, and A is true, then B is true. (309)

Are they getting warmer? Perhaps, but at a snail's pace. The "holy grail" search for reductive or unidirectional causes is fruitless and only makes matters worse in terms of reification. With the discovery of neuroplasticity, dual causality, and epigenetics the landscape has changed completely and the call is for a completely different orientation and tools; namely, the recognition and utilization of the power of language. As Paula Caplan (1995) puts it:

> Furthermore, much of the time and energy that professionals who use the DSM invest in learning about and trying to apply its contents could be more usefully invested in such endeavors as paying careful, caring attention to what one's patients say and working, free from dogma, to understand and help them. (xviii)

Furthermore, as mentioned in the beginning of this book, the ICD classification system in the domain of mental health has all the same problems as the DSM: labels defined by sufficient "symptoms" combined with "functional impairment."

We now turn our attention to the organizing core of our linguistic constructions—metaphors.

EIGHT

Why This Is the Wrong Metaphor to Begin With

In the clinical reality of the modernist worldview a "chemical imbalance" is an essential truth, just as are "diagnoses." Constructions such as these, seen as essential or absolute realities, form the organizing center of gravity upon which the whole clinical edifice (language, practices, and institutions) stands. These realities appear obvious, just as real as the words you're reading on page or screen; and the actions and utterances of the agents of these realities (therapists, psychiatrists, social workers) follow lockstep. Moreover, because of the self-confirming and self-fulfilling nature of language systems, this social constructivist recognition can only be seen from outside of the current prevailing clinical paradigm, that is, from the vantage point of postmodernism, neuroscience, and outcome studies.

Reductionist neuroscience brought us the "chemical imbalance." In his 1965 paper "The Catecholamine Hypothesis of Affective Disorders" Joseph J. Schildkraut (1965, 509) observed that his subjects classified as "having depression" showed lower levels of a class of neurotransmitter called catecholamines. Likewise with "schizophrenia" and excess dopamine (Baumeister and Francis, 2002). The stage was set for the "chemical imbalance" theory.

The point is that science uses metaphor all the time in its attempt to understand the world. In his book *I Is an Other: The Secret Life of Metaphor and How It Shapes the Way We See the World,* James Geary (2011) writes:

> Scientists and inventors compare two things: what they know and what they don't know. The only way to find out about the latter is to investigate the ways it might be *like* the former. And whenever we explore how one thing is *like* another, we are in the realm of metaphorical thinking. (loc. 226)

Furthermore, science and culture in general confuse metaphor with essential reality all the time. The reification from figurative metaphor to literal "truth" is part and parcel of the evolution of language as well as science. Metaphors die only to give rise to literal language. Geary (2011) continues:

> One of the ironies of etymology is that the less conscious we are of a metaphor as a metaphor, the more literal it becomes, a paradox observed by Nelson Goodman: "With progressive loss of its virility as a figure of speech, a metaphor becomes not less but more like literal truth. What vanishes is not its veracity but its vivacity." (loc. 452)

Far from blasphemy, to say the "chemical imbalance" is a metaphor, and not literal truth, is to say it's a routine product of science. And to say that the "chemical imbalance" metaphor has died and become *seeming* literal truth is to say that through its institutional usage it has become reified and has otherwise lived the typical life cycle of all metaphors. Science (or the pharmaceutical industry) may not be so quick to claim this inevitable fallibility: the "map" (or metaphor) is not the territory. But this represents science's reluctance to give up the certainty of its, often egoistically invested, old metaphors and venture into new metaphors and paradigms. In other words, "routine science" becomes institutionalized and its truths or "knowledge" are protected by virtue of the will to power.

METAPHORS WE LIVE BY[1]

It's important to see the metaphoric basis of science, knowledge, and everyday language because they insidiously determine what we see and don't see, what we attend to and don't attend to, what we say and don't say, what problems are legitimate and which are not, and most importantly—as far as "psychotherapy" is concerned—how we feel and don't feel. In the words of George Lakoff and Mark Johnson (1980):

> We have found . . . that metaphor is pervasive in everyday life, not just in language but in thought and action. Our ordinary conceptual system, in terms of which we both think and act, is fundamentally metaphorical in nature. . . . The concepts that govern our thought are not just matters of intellect. They also govern our everyday functioning, down to the most mundane details. Our concepts structure what we perceive, how we get around in the world, and how we relate to other people . . . our conceptual system is not something we are normally aware of. In most of the things we do every day, we simply think and act more or less automatically along certain lines. Just what these lines are is by no means obvious. One way to find out is by looking at language. Since communication is based on the same conceptual sys-

> tem that we use in thinking and acting, language is an important source of evidence for what that system is like.

Metaphors determine how we see the world and, accordingly, how we respond to the world. We've all heard antioxidants neutralize free radicals (those little devils in our bodies that break down DNA and cell walls) that cause aging—booming the nutritional supplement industry. Antioxidants are to us as preservatives are to cereal—the more the better! Can't you just imagine it? However in 2013 a *Scientific American* article "The Myth of Antioxidants" (Moyer, 2013) demonstrated how the situation is far more complex and that free radicals are essential for health and longevity; and that, in fact, many antioxidant supplements are linked to cancer. This myth started with Linus Pauling's—with his Nobel Prize celebrity status—obsession with vitamin C. Similarly, we have the cholesterol myth (Sinatra and Bowden, 2012). So we can see how the masses are swayed with seemingly sensible-sounding metaphors.

Far from being restricted to poetry, postmodern thinkers maintain that metaphor is the basis for thought and action. Moreover, our common, everyday language is replete with unrecognized metaphor, yet, unaware it determines our actions. Paul H. Thibodeau and Lera Boroditsky (2011) put it as follows:

> We find that metaphors can have a powerful influence over how people attempt to solve complex problems and how they gather more information to make "well-informed" decisions. Our findings shed further light on the mechanisms through which metaphors exert their influence, by instantiating frame-consistent knowledge structures, and inviting structurally-consistent inferences. Interestingly, the influence of the metaphorical framing is covert: people do not recognize metaphors as an influential aspect in their decisions.

"Metaphors exert their influence by instantiating frame-consistent knowledge structures, and inviting structurally-consistent inferences"; in other words, a metaphor acts as an organizing worldview, a substrate, upon which all kinds of other presuppositions, inferences, language, and practices evolve and depend. An entire profession, research and clinical reality, is the accrual of "knowledge structures" that emanate from a few poorly conceived metaphors: "chemical imbalance" and "psychiatric diagnoses." If the "diagnostic" and "chemical imbalance" metaphoric basis of these fundamental assumptions and presuppositions is wrong (outdated) then the entire edifice collapses.

In mental health the organizing metaphors of "chemical imbalances" and psychiatric "diagnoses" give rise to frame-consistent clinical language and practice. The ideas of "assessing a client" or "developing a treatment plan" or "case management" all revolve around the clinical metaphor. It's easy to see how the clinical roles of professional and patient are scripted down to the level of body postures and tone of voice.

But like some insidious straightjacket the perceptions of and responses to clients are correspondingly circumscribed. Attitude is everything and a clinical, deficit-based, pathologizing worldview brings forth the corresponding attitude which positions persons as broken, incapable, fragile, and (in some metaphysical way) diseased.

Referring back to the Thibodeau and Boroditsky quote above: "Interestingly, the influence of the metaphorical framing is covert: people do not recognize metaphors as an influential aspect in their decisions." Language systems contain metaphors and therefore metaphors are part of the fabric of subjectivity and as such their influence is pervasive, insidious, and has profound consequences. Perhaps it is part of human nature (i.e., human subjectivity) to make entire institutional edifices based on illusory premises. George Eliot wrote in *Middlemarch* (1874/2003):

> For we all of us, grave or light, get our thoughts entangled in metaphors, and act fatally on the strength of them.

THE BRAIN AS MACHINE

In the medical model the brain is seen as acting in a fixed, mechanical, and unidirectional way to cause emotions, behavior, and thinking—like a pancreas produces insulin. And, as the story goes, the brain can have neurotransmitters out of balance like a pancreas can fail to produce sufficient amounts of insulin. At this point we're left—as "patients"—to the beneficence of the pharmaceutical industry (see *Saving Normal: An Insider's Revolt against Out-of-Control Psychiatric Diagnosis, DSM-5, Big Pharma, and the Medicalization of Ordinary Life* by Allen Frances, former chairperson for the DSM-IV, 2013a).

The story of how we've come to view human behavior reductively is interesting. During the seventeenth and eighteenth centuries humanity was enamored with reason and science. Reason was shown to have so many useful applications that it was thought that everything, including the human body, the human psyche, even God, could be completely understood in terms of rational analysis.

René Descartes's (1637/1998) *Discourse on Method* explained that to understand a complex phenomenon we simply need to break it down into its component parts and analyze how the parts interact to produce the observed phenomenon. Isaac Newton extrapolated from his law of motion that the universe was like a giant clock with parts interacting according to rational principles. The reductionistic (Descartes) and mechanistic (Newton) explanatory methods turned out to be so powerful (in terms of explanation, prediction, and invention) that science and medicine assumed that they could apply reason to explain all human behavior and human experience. This is the foundation of modern medicine and psychiatry. Behavior problems and human emotional suffering are analyzed into the smallest component parts (neurotransmitters and neurons) and analyzed as to their interactions (synapses and neural networks). In essence, psychology treats people with difficulty living as if they were broken machines, forever looking to fix or replace the broken parts (chemical imbalances). This works fine with simple systems, but with complex systems this is completely inadequate. This misapplication of reductive science where it doesn't belong (also economics) is called *scientism*.

BETTER SCIENCE, BETTER METAPHORS

As scientific progress goes, the trend has been the better the scientific methods of observation, the better the metaphor in terms of its correspondence with nature and its explanatory power. The atom was once thought of as infinitesimally small hard particles (e.g., like marbles) packed together to form macroscopic objects, later a tiny planet (nucleus) with satellites (electrons) revolving around it, and finally, something almost entirely composed of space whose composite "particles" have both wave and particulate qualities, whose position can only be known probabilistically, whose nature changes upon observation. With new metaphors come new paradigms and possibilities.

As we've already noted, the chemical imbalance metaphor was both cause and effect of the reductionist approach to understanding the human brain. *Reductionist neuroscience,* à la Descartes, utilized powerful imaging techniques to establish the essential biochemical nature of the "disease" as compared with "normal." Notwithstanding the issue of holistic medicine, reductive science seems to work better with other organs of the body, but it is wholly insufficient when looking at the organ of adaptation, the human brain.

Complexity neuroscience, the neuroplasticity branch of neuroscience, developed out of examining whole brain changes that occur as a result of the brain's "rising to the occasion" in the face of challenging environmental conditions and repetitive changes in thought, language, perception, and behavior. This alone should clue you into how much of a better fit complexity neuroscience—as opposed to reductive neuroscience—is with helping people deal with the challenge of life and themselves. Complexity neuroscience also recognizes the human brain in its social context; the mind, brain, and relationships united as one in the flow of energy and information.

Luckily for us neuroscience, using powerful imaging techniques, has discovered that the brain is a complex system with emergent properties where, in addition to the parts affecting the whole, the whole affects the parts. The human brain like other complex systems is irreducible: the emergent properties of the whole (language, thinking, subjectivity, behavior) cannot be understood by an analysis of the parts (neurons, synapses, and neurotransmitters). Much like the wetness of water cannot be studied by an analysis of the separate elements hydrogen and oxygen.

When we do study the whole brain in its role of adaptation to the environment we discover there is dual causality or, said another way, the human brain is reflexively related to behavior and thinking (which includes language). Emotions change indirectly through behavior and thought change. This is the basis of neuroplasticity.

To reiterate: In their groundbreaking introduction of neuroplasticity to the public *The Mind and the Brain: Neuroplasticity and the Power of Mental Force*, Jeffrey Schwartz and Sharon Begley (2002, 90) describe how mindfulness and cognitive behavioral therapy produced the same brain scan image changes as powerful psychotropic drugs (the placebo issue aside). As was amply illustrated in chapter 2 ("Neuroplasticity"), other researchers have since verified that higher holistic brain functions (thinking coordinated with behavioral changes) produce changes in lower emotional centers. The brain, like all complex systems, is self-regulating.

We now recognize that both research and commonsense observation tell us that with changes in language, perspective, and behavior the human brain changes. As we will see in the chapter on postmodern coaching, problem redescription (changes in language, thinking, and perspective) and acquisition of new skills (changes in behavior) are recursively related (mutually influencing one another) and each requires deliberate and repetitive practice. Our emotions change as a result of this process. In other words, the new neuronal networks improve both our subjectively felt experience and our performance on the playing field of life. More adaptive neuronal networks replace less adaptive neuronal networks—in terms of both perspective and practice. There's plenty of cortex. Do we need to know the exact neuronal machinery involved in such changes? Does it matter if we both feel better and perform better?

The point is that the new frontier of intersubjective space—the source of these neuronal changes in psychotherapy—has hardly begun to be explored. In other words, the practical implications of the discovery of neuroplasticity have to be worked out in practice. New findings in complexity neuroscience are gravy at this point.

Thus the disease model—itself a metaphor—breaks down with the recognition of the brain as a complex system, neuroplasticity, and epigenetics.

CONSTRUCTIVISM VERSUS REALISM

This postmodern/complexity neuroscience perspective is consistent with both the constructivists (truth as interpretation; language as creational) and realists (truth as correspondence with the physical world; language as representational) camps of philosophy. With better observational tools—positron emission tomography (PET), functional magnetic resonance imaging (fMRI), etc.—we've discovered the physical "reality" of the brain is different than what we previously thought. We have to consider the human brain as a whole, in its relational context, and in the context of its adaptive capabilities; that is, from the perspective of complexity (versus reductive) neuroscience. Neuroplasticity is a model of the brain that better corresponds with nature (physical reality), has better explanatory power, and, as we will see, produces far better results.

On the other hand, the more realistic picture of the brain given to us by complexity neuroscience has helped explain how our realities are socially constructed. Our higher-level brain functions can network words and symbols in such a way as to produce different realities. The significance of subjectivity was rediscovered with the tools of objectivity. The question is no longer about the reality of neuroplasticity, but how best to bring it about. When it comes to psychotherapy, I believe the best answer to date is intersubjectivity and redescription.

BRAIN-BEHAVIOR REFLEXIVITY

The language of psychiatry is based on the assumption of one-way causality and the brain as a mechanistic or simple system. This illness model assumes that "chemical imbalances" in the brain cause psychiatric "symptoms." The "symptoms" tend to, in some rough way, form characteristic clusters (in statistical analyses of larger populations) which then are given a label, commonly referred to as a "diagnosis." The "diagnosis" is one of many possible under the major umbrella "mental illness." Furthermore, a person labeled with a "mental illness" takes on a patient identity.

The important point is that *one-way causality* is a foundational presupposition embedded in the language and practice of psychiatry; and the patient identity is a natural consequence of this inadequate and outdated metaphor referred to as the "chemical imbalance." This is true no matter how "client centered," "recovery oriented," "wellness focused," or "strength based" a program is.

On the other hand, complexity neuroscience has long recognized the brain as a complex organ capable of emergent properties (mind, consciousness, thought, intentionality, etc.). Danielle Bassett and Michael Gazzaniga (2011) describe this brain-behavior/thinking reflexivity:

> Emergence is characterized by a higher-level phenomenon stemming from a lower system level; that is, emergence is upward. However, an important property of the brain, as opposed to some other complex systems, is that emergent phenomena can feedback to lower levels, causing lower level changes through what is called downward causa-

> tion. The combination of upward emergence and downward causation suggests a simple bidirectionality or more nuanced mutual complementarity that adds to the complexity of the system, and underscores the fact that the emergence of mental properties cannot be understood using fundamental reductionism. (200)

The ability of the emergent properties of the higher centers of the brain to influence the chemistry of the lower levels is highly dependent on attention, thought, language, and context.

The "chemical imbalance" idea is not a truth. It's simply a metaphor created to try to explain emotional difficulties and to suggest a solution (add chemicals to put our brain into "balance")—convenient to certain industries. To what extent the chemical solution works is debatable; certainly in some cases, questionable in many others. Irving Kirsch, associate director of the Program in Placebo Studies and a lecturer in medicine at the Harvard Medical School, in his investigation of U.S. Food and Drug Administration unpublished research files (obtained only through use of the Freedom of Information Act) concluded that 80 percent of the improvement with antidepressant medication was placebo effect (Kirsch, 2002)! What we should be looking at is the consequences of the metaphor that has been misstated to the profession and public as scientific truth.

Moreover, the controversy as to whether or not "chemical imbalances" cause "mental illness" is moot. There's no question that there are *neural correlates* to all behavior, emotion, and thought; but the breakthrough in neuroplasticity is that repetitive alteration in behavior, language, and thought changes the physical structure of the brain. Said another way, the brain is *reflexively* related to behavior and thought (which includes language). The Dalai Lama's foreword to Sharon Begley's *Train Your Mind, Change Your Brain* (2008) puts it this way:

> Buddhist practitioners familiar with the workings of the mind have long been aware that it can be transformed through training. What is exciting and new is that scientists have now shown that such mental training can also change the *brain*. Related to this is evidence that the brain adapts or expands in response to repeated patterns of activity, so that in a real sense the brain we develop reflects the life we lead. (viii)

Using the language of psychiatry, as far as the human brain is concerned—like no other organ of the human body—if you change the "symptoms" (behaviors, thinking, and language) you cure the "disease" (the associated neural network)! Again, emotions are always dealt with indirectly through thought and behavior change.

The reflexive relationship between the brain and "the life we lead" is even more intimate and connected when we consider the proposition that the mind *is* the brain. In other words, our physical brain is changing on some level when we are mindful, listening, reading, or simply experiencing. Simply by "paying attention" to something our brain is physically changing.

Colin McGinn (1999), a noted contemporary philosopher, points out that our separation of conscious mental states (e.g., thought, feeling, intentionality) from the material brain is a product of historical contingency. McGinn noted that René Descartes's dualism famously separated the mind from the brain (or matter) as distinct realities. With later scientific progress this dualism became modified to the assertion that the brain *produces* the mind. McGinn (1999) claims that the best neuroscience to date indicates that the mind *is* the brain:

> Neural processes are conscious processes. Nor is it merely that conscious processes are an aspect of neural processes; it is rather that there is nothing more to a conscious state than its neural correlate. (18)

Thus, how we constitute our mind with thought, language, concept, and metaphor becomes extremely important in terms of the brain's ability to change itself.

MIND, BRAIN, RELATIONSHIP REFLEXIVITY

As is mentioned throughout this book, our subjectivity (or mind) is intersubjectively constituted. Our mind, and therefore brain, is a product of our communications with other human beings. Daniel Siegel (2012, 26–27) refers to the mind, brain, and relationships as a triangular unity. All three elements mutually influence one another. This has been a theme throughout this book, and rather than restate everything I want to emphasize what intersubjectivity means in this context. Intersubjectivity is that sacred space where the flow of energy and information is highly focused, highly individualized, and made highly accessible. The therapist in this way is a conduit that adjusts to the client's frame of reference in such a way that key information in the form of human wisdom can be communicated. We're kind of a "universal adapter" for the flow of human intelligence.

COMPLEX SYSTEMS, EMERGENT PROPERTIES, AND THE MALLEABILITY OF HUMAN SUBJECTIVITY

We've talked about the brain being a complex system capable of emergent properties, wherein the higher centers of the brain feed back and alter or subsume lower centers of the brain, but what does this mean? Let's start by taking a look at the physical structure of the human brain.

The cerebral cortex, the outer layer of neural tissue (less than a quarter of an inch thick, surrounding the entire brain)—often referred to as the "gray matter"—is the higher center of brain function. In all mammals the cerebral cortex acts to integrate sensory data, instinctual drives, and memory in order to make more flexible and context-dependent "decisions." The human brain differs from other mammalian brains in that it has a greatly expanded and elaborated cerebral cortex. The increased complexity of the human cerebral cortex, including the addition of the somewhat thicker prefrontal cortex, is the source of higher brain functions such as consciousness, language, thought, awareness, perception, planning, and decision-making. Analogous to its physical location outside the rest of the brain it has the capacity to put the rest of the brain function, including itself, into perspective. It's able to "observe" the operations of the entire brain of which it encases, for example our animal instincts.

Without this cortical "observational" platform other animals are simply run by their instincts (i.e., the rest of the brain, namely, the brain stem and limbic systems) with no awareness of it. Mammals having a simplified cortex are capable of rudimentary learning and decisions, but are still dominated by their instincts.

Though all humans are fitted with the hardware, the higher brain functions are dependent on training—language and social experience. We've all observed young children go through the painful process of gaining gradual self-awareness and self-control over their otherwise "animal-like" impulses generated by limbic and brain stem systems—the "rat" and "reptile" brains, respectively. As is the current state of human affairs that alternative to our animal instincts is the culture imposed on us through the forceful and repetitive use of language by parents, other caretakers, and the social world as a whole. Progressively, through interactions with representatives of the culture (our caregivers), the cultural world, predicated in language, comes into existence. Through this sometimes brutal process of enculturation we internalize this linguistically channeled alternative force; Sigmund Freud called this (languaged this as) the "super ego."

With language and culture "the world" appears. We awaken from the unconscious experience of instinct into a "world" of social expectations and demands. Out of the darkness of instinct we emerge into the illusions of subjectivity. However, subjectivity is not random; it is a linguistically constituted coordination of action with the social world. Subjectivity is a testament to cultural evolution's recognition of the value of cooperative living to the human species as a whole.

Of course, as the attachment theorists will attest, this process of intersubjective attunement integrated with the truths, dictates, and expectations of culture is a process fraught with difficulty and error. Thank goodness for Donald Winnicott's (1975) concept of "good enough parenting." The end result is a greater or lesser degree of enculturation which includes a greater or lesser ability to occupy roles. This is our "rough and ready" answer to nature's aggressive, anxious, and sexual impulses.

Moreover, culture and subjectivity in general are a sublimation (to use another of Freud's terms) or channeling of these instincts into more socially acceptable expressions. The resulting world we inhabit is a function of this childhood conditioning or childhood default narrative (our infamous life "story"). The sublimation of nature's instincts into culture is the prime a priori example of higher levels of brain functioning altering or subsuming lower levels of brain functioning.

Needless to say, the nature of subjectivity varies from culture to culture, time period to time period, family to family, and person to person. If subjectivity is ice cream, the variety of human cultures is the variety of flavors. Subjectivity is our interface with the world and *is* our world. Consequently, as the French author Anaïs Nin (1961, 124) quotes the Jewish Talmud: "We do not see things as *they are*, we see them as *we are*." We project a world and then mistake it for objective reality. Ernst Cassirer (1963) was first to point out that with human beings even sense perception is always linguistically mediated; in other words, "seeing" things is interpreting them; the meaning given to things allows us to "see" them. Remember the 180 types of snow; we don't "see" them (distinguish them) until we label each of them and ascribe meaning to each (good for packing, good for sled driving, etc.). We move from the oneness of infancy to a world made of words or distinctions, increasingly refined, differentiated, and useful.

Unfortunately aside from a few intellectuals, the recognition and profundity of subjectivity is unknown, despite it being the sine qua non of what makes us human. Of course, on a superficial level, personal experience and psychology will tell us that we operate out of a point of view and that our interpretations of our life circumstances are, well, subjective. But the degree to which our entire worldview is predicated in language and tradition cannot be overstated and has only begun to be appreciated in postmodern circles.

The postmodern philosophical movement began with Friedrich Nietzsche's perspectivism—the idea that there are no absolutes, no "thing in itself," no metaphysical world; but instead all there is is perspective. Putting it simply, Nietzsche asserted, "There are no facts, only interpretations." Keeping in mind how interpretation and subjectivity are constituted in language, Martin Heidegger (1959/1971) and Ludwig Wittgenstein (1922), added the primacy of language: "We don't use language, language uses us," and "The limits of my language means the limits of my world," respectively. Søren Kierkegaard (1846/1992) proclaimed, "Subjectivity is truth." Michel Foucault (1983) emphasized how knowledge and language are instruments of power. Subjectivity is real and it is the purview of both postmodernism and complexity neuroscience.

From this point of view we can definitively say that subjectivity/language is *the* emergent property of the human brain. Moreover, we know from psychotherapy, other transformational modalities, and common observational sense that subjectivity is malleable. We change. Our view of the world changes as we live and experience life and relationships. Complexity neuroscience has simply demonstrated that our change has neural correlates. In a sense, complexity neuroscience has freed us from the hypnotic trance of science as inappropriately applied to human beings (aka scientism)—its categories, mechanistic interpretation of human beings, obsession with efficiency and technology—into the art of living. Being science obsessed we had to have science (i.e., cognitive science) tell us where its limitations lie, that is, in the domain of the human spirit and human behavior.

Of course, our enculturation is far from perfect and our routine, automatic, and often inflexible ways of interpreting and responding to the world are often insufficient and sometimes counterproductive. In many ways in the beginning we persist in using the tools we have despite their ineffectiveness—doing the same thing and expecting different results. Eventually, out of emotional pain and/or performative difficulties, we seek help. We've entered the path of personal/spiritual growth or human transformation and I contend *that this applies to all humans*. In other words, we need not make creative, sensitive, imaginative, or emotional people into "patients" in need of "treatment." Personal or spiritual growth—human transformation—is for all!

Whereas culture dealing with instinct involved the neocortex dealing with the limbic and brain stem systems (aka untempered emotional centers), the neocortex as mentioned above has the capacity to contextualize, or gain perspective on, itself. The human brain is able to acquire new perspectives and new interpretations which can alter its feelings and actions. This is the basis of both cultural evolution as well as individual transformation. As part of its maturation the brain is able to see everything it "knows" as interpretation, that multiple conflicting perspectives can coexist, that context determines the best interpretation, and that thinking involves considering and integrating multiple points of view. In other words, in support of adaptation, the thickened neocortex allows us to occupy new vantage points, to question our assumptions, to redescribe, to reinterpret, and finally to enter new paradigms of thought and action.

The pliability of subjectivity in the service of human transformation comes in many forms. Socratic inquiry and behavioral experiments in cognitive behavioral science open up new ways of interpreting our challenging situations. Psychodynamic and object-relations therapy facilitate corrective emotional experiences that liberate us from our childhood default narratives. Postmodern therapies allow for leveraging individual temperaments, redescribing life circumstances, supporting self-determination, and altering personal narratives and identities—all free, relatively speaking, from the rigid modernist truths, categories, and power relations. Mindfulness skills change our relationship to thought, feeling, sensation, and even perception—allowing us to observe these phenomena. Human wisdom as revealed in literature, philosophy, history, poetry, personal/spiritual growth movements, religion, and other postmodern-based human transformational movements can alter our view of the world, ourselves, and our feelings, thoughts, and actions.

Finally, free from the reified metaphysical constructs of the clinical vocabulary we're finally in a position to leverage the very source of the transformative power of the human brain: language. Language and metaphor can emerge in our intersubjective engagement with others and dramatically alter our way of being in the world. Again, new perspective and new skills require repetitive practice and an appreciation for incremental change in order for new neural circuits to form, constituting what we might otherwise call a "second nature."

Our search for emotional well-being, meaning, and better performance on the playing field of life requires that we find increasingly better subjective frameworks. Alternative interpretations, relanguaging, and redescription result in new experimental action. The action, in turn, feeds back into the experimental perspective. The expansion of our subjectivity is from lower to higher order, the building of greater and greater context and performative flexibility. New emergent properties subsume pre-existing emergent properties as the channeling of instinct becomes more refined, complex, and socially responsible. Civilization and cultural evolution are built on the emergent properties of the brain as a complex system.

Complexity neuroscience has done its job. Given the universe of possibilities that it has opened up to us—intersubjective space and the malleability of mind/brain—complexity neuroscience is irrelevant to those of us concerned with its practical applications in the domain of human transformation—for now at least. This is true especially in light of the fact that neuroscience's scientific (academic) vocabulary and framework continue to blind us to the artful vocabulary, dialogic skills, and worldly perspectives required to enter intersubjective space and leverage it in terms of human transformation. We need to focus on the incredible vast and new landscape that complexity neuroscience has opened up to us—the art of human transformation. Else, we will continue to confuse the finger for what it is pointing to.

NEUROPLASTICITY IS HARD WORK

Moreover, neuroplasticity and complexity are better metaphors because they imply the importance of mobilizing client energy, focus, attention, initiative, responsibility, experimental perspective, decisiveness, learning mindset, and committed action. Employing a metaphor of disease—where the fundamental root of the problem lies in abnormal brain physiology—when brain change requires so much focused attention, commitment, hard work, practice, persistence, responsibility, and the ability to bounce back—completely short-circuits this arduous change process.

The way the issue is framed makes all the difference; literally different realities! The right framework reflects neuroplasticity. The old framework of disease casts the person in the role of a passive, insecure, incompetent, dependent, fragile "patient." The new framework of neuroplasticity and coaching implies boldness, confidence, competence, interdependence, and strength. Importantly, you can't conclude anything about the potential capability of the people, family members, clients, or friends because the helping efforts heretofore have been embedded in the pathologizing, deficit-based clinical worldview—even if unstated or unawares. Furthermore, the clinical world disappears when we understand the "chemical imbalance" as a metaphor and not an essential or absolute reality.

The emphasis on hard work and practice can't be overstated. Even if Irving Kirsch (2002) is correct and as much as 80 percent of the effect of antidepressant medication is placebo effect, the placebo effect reflects the power of belief (Lipton, 2008, 110). And if you're going to stop taking psychiatric medications you're going to need perspectives and practices in place to help you deal with yourself and your circumstances successfully. To reiterate, this book is not a call to stop taking psychiatric medications, it's a call to add the effort of personal and spiritual transformation to your program for well-being.

A METAPHOR CONSISTENT WITH WHAT WORKS

The overwhelming consensus in the profession, based on empirical evidence, is that the therapeutic alliance is the highest predictor of success in psychotherapy. As we've seen, the therapeutic alliance (outcome research emphasis) and intersubjectivity (interpersonal neurobiology and attachment theory emphasis) are two sides of the same coin, both of which are highly dependent on (1) the relational stance of unconditional positive regard, accurate and felt empathy, and therapist congruence; (2) the dialogic skill of moment-by-moment presence, receptivity, and responsiveness of the therapist; and (3) redescriptive (or interpretive) resonance or fit. As mentioned before, often we combine (1) and (2) leaving us with (1) intersubjectivity and (2) interpretive resonance. With this in mind, the choices of metaphor are between "chemical imbalance" (psychiatric diagnoses) and neuroplasticity.

The chemical imbalance metaphor is the organizing center of the entire symptom-obsessed, disease-focused clinical worldview. The hardened categories/metaphors/realities of the clinical world blind us to the subtleties and nuances of our client's world. Concepts, metaphors, and words determine what we "see," and what we see determines how we think, feel, and respond. What does a therapist/psychiatrist see? They see clients not as they are, but as the therapist/psychiatrist is. They see "hyperverbalness," "internal distraction," "impaired judgment," "poor insight," "mania," "depressed mood," "unstable self-image," inability to regulate emotions, incompetence, "flat affect," fragility, "narcissism," "low self-esteem"—all of which lead to "seeing" a psychiatric "diagnosis." They see these things not because they are objectively there, but because they've been trained in a particular vocabulary that interprets people through a particular set of metaphors. This is the culture of psychiatry. Moreover, "symptoms," "diagnoses," and other clinical "treatment" systems derive from a more general normative worldview with its associated normative templates (or standards of what is considered "normal").

Normative templates, by way of personal prejudices or "clinical judgments," preclude us from non-judgmentally and authentically participating in another person's subjective world. Unconditional positive regard, accurate empathy, authenticity require the absence of normative judgments. Other relational skills such as aligning with goals and preferences, taking serious and addressing concerns, privileging the person's preferences and choices, and real-time moment-to-moment pivots in responsiveness are similarly precluded by the clinical worldview.

The subtle distinctions of the dialogic art of psychotherapy are hidden by the bulky, clumsy, and totalizing clinical categories. The client's emotive and non-verbal responses tell us how close we are to their experience and whether or not our redescriptions *take hold* with them. This dialogic art form is very dynamic and collaborative. The search for fitting and better adaptive interpretations/descriptions is a very nuanced, trial-and-error process that takes place within the client's frame of reference.

The disease model is *incompatible* with the not-knowing, non-normative, non-judgmental stance required for multiperspective receptivity, interpretive flexibility, and timely responsiveness. In the clinical world the therapist is knowing (assessing and diagnosing), operating out of a normative frame (a diagnosis implies abnormality), and judgmental (the disease model implies a negative connotation). Recall that this clinical reality does not show up as one interpretation among many, it appears as real as the chair you're sitting in as you read this. This is the way we experience our enculturation (subjection). Moreover, when we step outside of this clinical reality we enter *the now* vis-à-vis our participation in the very dynamic world of subject-to-subject dialogue.

Fritz Perls, the founder of Gestalt therapy, used to say, "Lose your mind and come to your senses" (1969/1992, 16–17). Not that we could return to our pre-linguistic animal state, but we certainly have to drop the clinical vocabulary that would have us think we were objectively observing a person. Our interpretive framework should support our collaborative meaning making out of our here-and-now dialogic engagement with a person. Of course it follows that therapist training should be all about dialogic skill and the perspectives that support generative, collaborative dialogue and the production of useful descriptions and metaphors.

The client's inner world is revealed to us in very subtle non-verbal and verbal ways. The words they use, the inflections and tones, and in all the other subtle ways emotion is expressed in the body. Then there is the subtle recursive dance between the therapist's communications and actions and the client's responses. Again, the word is dynamic. This "becoming one with the client" (to use a Zen phrase) is completely fouled up when the therapist is *standing on* the deficit-based clinical reality. Believing is seeing. You literally can't see the client's world if you're seeing symptoms; this is how we're captured by language. In my experience this is true even of therapists who are striving to learn this method. As long as the clinical world is seen as a reality the client's reality will be elusive. Remember the difference between an improvisational musician and an automobile mechanic!

In the clinical world the therapist or doctor is the expert and the client is the non-expert. In some Procrustean fashion, the client is expected to comply with or accept what is offered. This is an inherently hierarchical relationship, not unlike a parent-child relationship. It should be abundantly clear that this precludes an adult-to-adult or subject-to-subject relationship where both client and professional participate in the co-creation of new possibilities. Where the client's world is just as valid as the therapist's or doctor's. Where privileging client choice is far more important than what might be thought of as the best, perhaps most rational or prudent, course of action to be taken. Where detailed explanation, redescription, and unprejudiced persuasion replace formulaic recommendation or directive; interpersonal skill replaces the authority of role, position, or title; choice replaces compliance. Where "failure" is just as good as "success"—both provide information to help us formulate our next move. Where life experience is the best teacher.

The roles, setting, language, rituals, and the entire institutional context—founded on an illusion—are as fabricated as any theatrical or Hollywood production. Recognizing that "all the world's a stage" we actually have creative control over the production. The hierarchical relationship is a construction embedded in the medical worldview. The call for expertise is greater than ever, only of a vastly different kind. From the postmodern point of view, the professional's expertise lies in his/her own transformative life experience and his/her dialogic skill in connecting and staying connected and in traversing the exciting world of the in-between, the world of intersubjectivity.

Like culture in general, metaphorically constituted linguistic frameworks are built with interconnected words, concepts, values, and practices; as such they compose a context. As we saw in chapter 5, the subjugating power of the context springs into existence with the utterance of one word, *any* word derived from that framework.

NOTE

1. Title from *Metaphors We Live By* by George Lakoff and Mark Johnson (1980).

III

A Fundamental Egalitarianism

NINE

The Creation of the Patient

As part of the rationalization, medicalization, bureaucratization, and institutionalization of the modern world, professions, institutions, and society promote mass ways of looking at and responding to people—i.e., people are put into categories. Like other arbitrary cultural practices they are simply passed down through communication, tradition, custom, convention, state sanction, and in the case of mental health, a very, very tenuous claim to scientific legitimacy. For example, the criminal justice system has no problem labeling people "criminals," "ex-cons," and "felons"—defining identities instead of simply addressing behaviors. And, of course, the people themselves participate in their own subjugation by using these labels on themselves. Irony of ironies, the criminal justice system creates *criminals* with their reckless use of language; the mental health system similarly creates *patients*. Again, the profundity of this only becomes clear from a vantage point—itself spoken into existence—from outside the prevailing institutions.

People with difficulties with living may be from time to time confused, emotionally disturbed, displaying counterproductive patterns of behavior, and behaviorally out of control, but it's only after repeated encounters with the clinical institution that they are scripted as patients. They're treated as "fragile," incompetent, manipulative, helpless, broken, dependent, "axis II," and sometimes as dangerous. The clinical vocabulary is deficit based and pathologizing. The mental health professionals "see," feel, think, and act through the lens of their vocabulary. They see "symptoms" that confirm the label and accordingly take the actions that follow in the medicalized vocabulary: assess, diagnose, treat, "psycho educate," case manage, triage. Linda Logan chronicled this very experience in her 2013 *New York Times Magazine* article:

> The moment the psych-unit doors locked behind me, I was stripped of my identity as wife, mother, teacher and writer and transformed into patient, room number and diagnosis. . . . I would try to talk to my doctors about my vanishing self, but they didn't have much to say on the subject. Instead they focused on whether I could make eye contact or how much expression I showed in my face.

Systems theorists have long been interested in relationship and communication. They realized that when we speak we "position" the "other." Role expectations and power relations (context) as well as words (content) are conveyed in all our communications. Referencing Gregory Bateson's work, Don Jackson (1965) concluded:

> Every message (communication bit) has both a content (report) and a relationship (command) aspect; the former conveys information about facts, feelings, experiences, etc., and the latter defines the nature of the relationship between the communicants. (8)

The mental health profession has completely ignored this crucial aspect of communication. The command aspect is conveyed in everything from tone of voice to body posture, what is said and how it is said, as well as the lack of dignity conveyed in paternalism or in the lack of excellent customer service in all its detailed manifestations. When people are not granted dignity nor treated with excellent customer service, what's really being communicated implicitly—the most powerful form of communication—is "you're not worthwhile," "you're inferior," "you're a loser," "your life, your feelings, your dreams, your concerns, your time, your well-being, your existence doesn't matter as much as other people's, or not at all." After this solid foundation has been set, then the pathologizing, infantilizing "treatment" begins. Stanley Kubrick might be interested in this. Again, this is what's happening at the level of right brain to right brain subjectivity, the subtleties of which remain undistinguished in the land of labels. Remember people see through their categories.

When you're under the illusion that you have an objective point of view and are performing an "intervention" *on* someone the influence you're *actually* having on the other person is ironic, that is, having the exact opposite effect as was intended. For example, in "telling" someone how to be independent you're actually positioning him or her as dependent. For them to "follow" your instructions on how to be "independent" would be to passively *comply* coming from a position of dependence. Similarly with the way people are scripted/positioned as patients whose job it is to *accept* their diagnosis and *comply* with treatment—superb training in submissiveness and passivity. This profound, life-altering influence is what's really happening—going completely unnoticed—beneath the surface of all the "sound and fury" of clinical jargon "signifying nothing."[1] Like some kind of macabre factory receiving the human raw materials as input and producing dependent patients as output—all the while, blinded by its self-confirming vocabulary, unable to see this.

As Friedrich Nietzsche discovered, what's going on beneath the workings of "polite," "civil," "rational," and "professional" relationships and institutions is the brutish will to power/knowledge/punish/control/define. Thomas Szasz aptly described this kind of sublimated natural selection:

> In the animal kingdom, the rule is eat or be eaten; in the human kingdom, define or be defined. (1973, 20)

The ritual ceremony of definition (and subjection)—both of problem and identity—is called the psychological assessment. This is where the therapist or psychiatrist thinks s/he is neutrally or objectively observing the client. This is subject-to-object relating. This includes all the forms of assessment of all the theoretical orientations of psychology; including such forms as the "bio-psycho-social assessment" and psychological testing or simply doing an "assessment" for the purposes of "diagnosing." In all of these cases the pathologizing clinical categories constitute the lenses from which the client is viewed. The purpose to reduce the multifaceted, multidimensional, multicontextual, multi-identity person to a clinical category, trait, dynamic, personality type, or diagnosis—all of which purport to be true, legitimate essences as if they were somehow based in nature herself. Furthermore, saying a person "has schizophrenia" versus "is a schizophrenic" makes no difference. Labeling in the form of "has" or "is" is largely indistinguishable as labeling feeling, thinking, and mind are constitutive of identity. Does the phrase "elephant in a porcelain factory" mean anything to you?

The infamous "bio-psycho-social" assessment is a mechanic's dream, so very thorough. If we use all our interrogative and detective work in the assessment of all aspects of a client's life we will know the nature of the client's problem and where to intervene. If we create a passive, dependent, compliant, or resistant "patient" in the process so be it! The imposition of this bio-psycho-social grid is at the expense the relationship, alliance, and, of course, intersubjectivity—the most important factors in the success of psychotherapy. Instead, from this new postmodern and coaching framework we're interested in activating the independent agency and responsibility of the client by virtue of the unfolding and expansion of their subjectivity. It's an art form. We're not car mechanics, we don't have to solve every problem a client has. This is a highly leveraged and efficient way to work—a little goes a long way. This is more like homeopathy than surgery.

As we have seen and will continue to see throughout this book this mechanistic and reductionistic view of human beings defies both the new realities of complexity theory and neuroplasticity. By virtue of the power of language it is nothing but self-fulfilling of its categories and defeating of the very purpose of the professional relationship: change!

Furthermore, questions focusing on past trauma and abuse, histories of relationship and job failure, etc., all paint a picture of deficit and dysfunction. A feast for a diagnostically oriented clinician. But a disaster for the recipient. It's no surprise that one would walk away from such an "assessment" feeling broken, insecure, weak, incompetent, specimen-like, alienated, etc. You can't escape the inevitable fact that you get more of what you focus on and, as we have seen, reification through focus and labeling will see to it that the seeming-negative experiences/characteristics and the seeming-client deficits "discovered" in the "assessment" will be focused on in perpetuity.

As has been mentioned before, language, perspective, and action should support three things: (1) the relational stance of unconditional positive regard, accurate and felt empathy, and therapist congruence/authenticity; (2) the dialogic skill of moment-by-moment presence, receptivity, and responsiveness of the therapist; and (3) interpretive flexibility and range needed to facilitate interpretive resonance or fit. Past events (e.g., traumatic experiences) and current difficulties arise, when and if they do, in the space of intersubjectivity where they are artfully reinterpreted in the service of problem dissolution and/or constructive action in the support of our client's commitments. In this new paradigm our vocabulary is changing from one of stasis by reifying made up entities and totalizing traits or propensities to one of change by using words, metaphors, language, concepts that facilitate change, committed action, and possibility.

The "mechanic" in his/her detective (i.e., assessment, diagnostic, and psychological-issues) modes may win a few battles at the cost of losing the war. The creation of the patient is what we call iatrogenic illness—"illness" created in the attempt to heal.

When celebrities like Jane Pauley, Mel Gibson, or Brooke Shields "come out of the closet" and reveal they have a "mental illness" they've simply succumbed to being defined vis-à-vis participating in their own subjugation. The ritual of accepting the clinical language is traditionally thought of as a necessary preliminary to "treatment"; in a very ironic use of the word, considered "good insight." As if being defined is not such a bad thing—a principle of "stigma" busting. A real act of courage would be to stand *against* being defined in the first place, to say we don't need pathologizing labels in order to participate in the transformative narrative of humankind, find our unique creative contribution to the world, and to thrive (with or without "pills"). The only condition we suffer from is the human condition—we all need help.

Not to be too hard on the mental health profession, this is true in general in human relations at this point in our development. There is a pervasive irony in human relationships. Our life story positions/characterizes others (as "bad," "incompetent," "lazy," "untrustworthy," "dangerous," etc.) then all our attempts to influence them are based from this presupposition about them. We spend a lifetime fulfilling self-fulfilling prophecies. The relationships in mental health are no exception to this tragic reality of human existence.

Needless to say the meanings and connotations of *"the patient"* role are debilitating. The presuppositions of the role include the cause of my problem is a chemical imbalance and the doctor is there to assess and balance out my brain chemistry using psychiatric medications; I'm fragile; I'm not normal; the professionals know better than me; someday I hope to "get better" (or "recover"); and I have to take these medications the rest of my life (forever fearful of a relapse). Their "script" (their actual speaking) is replete with such phrases as "my medication," "my doctor" and "my diagnosis is (or "I have") _________." The patient is symptom, diagnosis, medication, and deficit focused—what else would you expect? It's in the script!

When it comes to human beings, connotations (implied meanings of a word) are far more influential that denotations (a literal definition of a word). Denotation is a product of definition and reason. Connotation is an image or feeling implied by a word. Denotatively a lion is "a large, tawny-colored cat that lives in prides, found in Africa and northwest India." Connotatively a lion represents courage and dignity. To say someone is a "patient," denotatively we mean "a person receiving medical treatment." This is bad enough in light of the paradigm of language, neuroplasticity, and personal responsibility. However, when we look at the connotation of a "patient" with "mental illness" we get a far worse picture. Paula Caplan (1995) puts it this way:

> When terms like abnormal or mentally ill are spoken, what kinds of images come to mind? Usually, images of difference and alienation, suggesting that "they" are not as competent, human, or safe to be around as the rest of "us." And often, "abnormal" and "mentally ill" are equated with "crazy," a label that calls forth images of someone who is out of control, out of touch with "reality," incapable of forming a good relationship, untrustworthy, quite possibly dangerous, and probably not worth one's attention, time, or energy. If such labeling had some positive effects, it might be worth risking the negative consequences for those who are labeled abnormal. (11)

Recall that because the clinical world seems objective (reflecting reification and an unwarranted link to scientific legitimacy) professionals that do recognize these effects view them as, though unfortunate, inevitable. One palliative is the antistigma campaign.

People who have problems in living—the nature versus nurture controversy, notwithstanding—eventually, with continued exposure to the clinical vocabulary, embody the script of the fragile, nearly helpless, medication-dependent, and insecure "patient." Perennially, self-consciously aware of themselves as "patients." In the medication-centered universe examples of medicalized (pathological) interpretations of normal or excessive reactions to challenging situations abound. The normal or excessive ups and downs of employment or being in relationships quickly get pathologized. Being overwhelmed or anxious at work is interpreted as "I'm having a panic attack." Having difficulty getting up in the morning (who doesn't) is viewed as depression kicking in again. Excitement will never be the same again now that it's been defined as mania (or for the more diagnostically sophisticated: hypomania). Normal frustration or justifiable anger is often met by (medicalized) others with "Have you been taking your medications?" Shery Mead and Cheryl MacNeil (2006) in their paper titled "Peer Support: What Makes It Unique?" poignantly illustrate this problem:

> Recovery in mental health has most often been defined as a process by which people labeled with mental illness regain a sense of hope and move toward a life of their own choosing. . . . While this definition on the surface seems obvious, what remains hidden is the extent to which people have gotten stuck in a medical interpretation of their experiences. With this stuckness comes a worldview in which one is constantly trying to deal with their perception of what's wrong with them instead of what's wrong with the situation. In other words, even if I have hope of moving into a better life, I have been taught to pay a lot of attention to my "symptoms." This interpretation of my experiences leaves me constantly on guard for what might happen to me should I start to get "sick." Even with recovery skills (learning to monitor my own symptoms), I find myself creating a life that is ultimately guided by something inherently wrong with me. With this understanding, I may continue to see myself as more fragile than most, and different than "normal" people. I then continue to live in a community as an outsider, no matter what goals I achieve. (7)

This reflexive and automatic tendency to ascribe our difficulties with living in the complex modern world (along with the associated disturbing emotions) to "chemical imbalances" or "diagnoses" or "unresolved childhood issues" perpetuates the eternally recurring retreat from life back into the arms of the medical professionals.

They say "there's no atheist in a foxhole"; similarly in those instances where our mettle is tested in life's challenges people subject to the "chemical imbalance" metaphor resort to their "chemical imbalance" or "condition" ("diagnosis") as the source of the difficulty—rather than to the absence of critical skills, perspectives, and experience. Predictably the patient identity asserts its authority in the cauldron and crucible of life. The resulting persistence of the problem creates the illusion of an unalterable physiological cause.

The new paradigm of neuroscience and neuroplasticity has something different to say about this. Because emotional-thought-behavior *patterns persist due to repetition* and systemic complementarity (i.e., being surrounded by, scripted by, and otherwise defined by infantilizing and pathologizing others) they seem to have a life of their own and they are easily, understandably, and, albeit mistakenly, interpreted by *the patient* as "a condition" *inside* him or her.

Enduring emotional-thought-behavior patterns have neuronal correlates and are products of habit. Neurons that fire together wire together. The more a thought, feeling, behavior, or interpersonal pattern is repeated, the more firmly entrenched is the neural network—and therefore, the more likely it is to fire off. Furthermore, these disturbing and counterproductive emotional and behavioral patterns are supported by our personality and personal narratives (they contextualize and justify our negative feelings), which are neuronal patterns as well. You can see how easily an enduring and counterproductive emotional-thought-behavior pattern could be mistaken as a physical illness and permanent "condition." The difference lies in the perspective taken, complexity neuroscience versus reductive neuroscience, respectively.

Complexity neuroscience considers the brain as a whole, in its social context, and in its adaptive role of responding to the demands from its environment with repetitive changes in thought, language, perception, and behavior. Repetition of thinking/feeling/behaving leads to the strengthening and persistence of patterns of neuronal activity—in a word, a habit. Altering our thinking/feeling/behaving with the right perspective and repetitive practice becomes the new pattern or habit.

Reductive neuroscience, on the other hand, looks at the smallest component parts (e.g., neurons, neurotransmitters, synapses), how they interact, and how they differ in "normal" versus "abnormal" brains, and how to add or subtract components in order to repair the mechanism. As far as psychiatry and reductive neuroscience are concerned the human brain is as static and fixed as our kidneys, thus persisting "mental problems" would indicate permanent physiological brain abnormality—the illusion of a "permanent illness."

Adding a little serotonin here or a little dopamine there may be helpful, but if we label the neural network that correlates with the undesirable thinking/feeling/behavior pattern an "illness" dealt with primarily with "balancing" pharmaceuticals, the self-fulfilling prophesy should be obvious: we never do the hard work to alter our behavior, language, thinking, and lifestyle (that would have reversed the "illness"—neuroplasticity!) and therefore become forever dependent on "medications" and live out the medication-dependent lifestyle (i.e., the patient). We learn to "live with our 'illness.'" Here's one representative example.

I once had a teenage client come to my office reporting he was depressed. During our session we began to identify a pattern of thinking/

behavior/feeling (a neural network) which led to hopelessness and entertaining suicide. He had a very predictable pattern of overextending himself that was somehow related to pleasing others, needing to be admired, craving excitement, and distracting himself from disturbing thoughts/emotions. This eventually led to being overwhelmed and despairing over "how hard life was" and "it could only get worse as I get older." During the session he disclosed that he was so depressed that he cut his wrists.

His father agreed to take him to a nearby hospital to have him evaluated for psychiatric hospitalization. The hospital kept him for a week. Upon our next session I attempted to pick up where we left off with the above-mentioned pattern. However, I noticed how excited he was that he "had depression." Having been medicalized he felt taken care of and that it was somebody else's responsibility to fix his problem (i.e., the psychiatrist's). All he had to do was take the medications as prescribed. Given how chronically stressed, overwhelmed, and over-responsible he was, it was almost predictable that the "patient" role would be quite appealing. The reification of "depression" and its attribution as causal agent—outside of his control—completely eclipsed our prior conversation about the series of events which led to his overwhelm and hopelessness.

To the untrained it's often easy to think that disturbing overwhelming feelings and impulses come out of nowhere and have a life of their own—as is characteristic of what one would think of as an "illness." This interpretation had gained ground while he was in the hospital. In the light of patienthood, the coaching work and required committed action appeared to him as just another responsibility. In the meanwhile, I responded to his talk of "depression" with "what you call 'depression'" in order to stay within his frame of reference while still staying true to mine (i.e., committed to not reifying "depression"). The next session I was able to share all this with him. He began to see how—though it required a lot of practice with attention, mindfulness, and committed action—he could nip this pattern in the bud and that he could control "what he called 'depression'" (aka the pattern) thus narrowly escaping from the jaws of a lifetime of patienthood.

This is not to discount genetic propensities, but, the brain being a complex malleable system, it is able to change, temper, or adapt to these propensities. There is a presupposition of genetic determinism in psychiatry: if you inherit certain genes you develop the "illness." Whether or not there are heritable genes that when expressed lead to "schizophrenia" or "bipolar disorder" may be relevant; but more important is our alteration of lifestyle, behavior, language, and thinking that improve our performance in life and support our subjective experience of well-being. To use Robert Wright's (1994) metaphor genes are like knobs on a stereo and intentional and repetitive changes in our behavior, language, and thinking tune these knobs—they alter the expression of those genes—especially when it comes to the incredibly malleable brain.

Bruce Lipton in his *Biology of Belief* (2008) has made it a matter of public record that our environment, lifestyle, habits, behavior, thinking, feeling alter the expression of our genes—this is the field of epigenetics. The call for a total wellness program—including nutrition, exercise, rewarding relationships/occupation/spiritual life/private life, and subjective stability—has never been greater. As far as psychotherapy goes, Richard Glass (2008), *noted researcher in evidence-based medicine* at the University of Chicago, summarizes the new consensus:

> Recent research in brain imaging, molecular biology, and *neurogenetics* has shown that psychotherapy changes brain function and structure. Such studies have shown that psychotherapy affects regional cerebral blood flow, neurotransmitter metabolism, *gene expression*, and persistent modifications in synaptic plasticity. (1589; my italics)

Amazingly, the human brain has the capacity to change both its wiring and its genetic expression but it all hinges on our determined, disciplined, and creative effort to change our thinking, behavior, feeling, habits, and lifestyle, which in turn, has everything to do with our perspective (our actions follow from how the world appears to us), which in turn, is a function of language. To label a propensity (e.g., a "diagnosis")—genetic or conditioned in childhood—is to ensure it as destiny. Furthermore with what we now know about neuroplasticity, epigenetics, and the power of language and expectation we need a patient identity like we need a hole in our head!

Epigenetics is a well-known fact in terms of the body as a whole, which of course includes the brain, so in this general way we know epigenetics is a factor in the expression of those genes that are involved in the functioning of the human brain. But do we need to wait—Laputin-like—for scientific proof of alteration of the expression of specific mental health–related genetic sequences in order to take advantage of this new knowledge? Like was the case with neuroplasticity (needing scientific proof to take advantage of what was obvious from commonsense experience), our theoretical ontology (dependence on science and its labels) would make us wait until epigenetics definitively proves that genetic propensities for mental and emotional issues are amenable to changes in environment, lifestyle, relationships, nutrition, exercise, thinking, language, perspective, and behavior in general. But isn't their benefit (genetically based or not) obvious already! Our theoretical ontology cripples our ability to experiment with lifestyle changes and learn from experience. Fritz Perls again, "lose your mind and come to your senses." How did so-called "primitive" pre-modern people make a pharmacy out of the rain forest? By their connection to nature (their experience in-the-world), their experimental (trial and error) efforts, their ability to make fine discriminations, and their use of language. Can we *now* learn from *our* experience and think for ourselves? This is the art of living.

Patienthood versus personhood is the choice we face in the medical arena as well. Wellness is hard won. Whether we have diabetes, heart disease, or gum disease we have the choice as to the illness/patient route or wellness/person path. The difference lies in personal responsibility. Lifestyle changes—including diet and exercise—have been shown to reverse diabetes and heart disease (Campbell and Campbell, 2006). But habits, absent a do or die medical concern, are hard to change; and the focus on lifestyle changes to promote and maintain wellness is a paradigm shift requiring coaching as well. The "patient"—an identity embedded in the "illness" paradigm—lives life without sufficient concern for long-term health consequences; in effect, putting all the responsibility for health repair and maintenance on the physicians and surgeons. It's easy to take pills or have treatment done to you; not so easy to change habits and lifestyle. The "person"—the identity associated with the wellness paradigm—takes responsibility for coming up with, through trial and error, lifestyle changes what will establish and maintain wellness.

I once had the good fortune of running into a dentist with some imagination when it comes to getting people to floss. Most dentists tell you something to the effect of the importance of flossing to get food dislodged that would otherwise cause gum disease. A simple prosaic and unimaginative appeal to reason. Alas, as David Hume put it, "Reason is the slave of passion." So it's not surprising that simple logic doesn't result in people flossing regularly. As my dentist was cleaning my teeth, she explained that it was most crucial to floss at least once a day, especially before bedtime. Poetically she waxed, "During the day saliva works its way through your mouth like a stream, generally moving along food debris out from between your teeth. At night the saliva flow greatly slows and your mouth becomes like a pond, stagnant water, friendly to the proliferation of all kinds of organisms." I cringed as I saw in my imagination swampy, foul-smelling, dark, mosquito-ridden pond water. I was cured. Since that moment I rarely miss nightly flossing.

Such an example shows not only the power of metaphors to influence behavior, but a crucial shift in roles, responsibility, and language toward wellness. The dentist for that moment of coaching empowered me to take responsibility for the health of my gums. It is a complete paradigm shift from doctor-to-patient "treatment" to subject-to-subject (adult-to-adult) empowerment. One could imagine a bevy of distinctions, metaphors, and strategies that could be employed to facilitate the repetitive practice needed to create the changes of habit (i.e., neuronal circuitry changes) necessary to realize dental wellness. Such a shift in locus of responsibility and alteration of habits is diametrically opposed to the patient identity. There's a reason insurance companies call them wellness coaches and not wellness therapists—connotatively coaching presumes competence and therapy presumes incompetence. Ironically, to date mental health "wellness" or "recovery" programs remain embedded in the "illness" paradigm.

From the perspective of neuroplasticity life's challenges are expected and utilized. The point is to rise to the occasion and learn from experience. The consequences of one project (win, lose, or draw) set up the next project. Through trial and error—forever on the lookout for what works and what doesn't work—we put ourselves in the right soil, with the right amount of light and moisture; the right job or career, the right neighborhood, the right relationships, the right hobbies. We tailor make our nurturing environment and lifestyle right down to the kind of pillows we use.

Life's difficulties when met with a less than satisfactory response are ideal coaching opportunities, of which we will speak of in the chapter on postmodern coaching. With all due respect to intersubjectivity, timing, collaboration, temperament, and incremental change, the postmodern coach's relational stance doesn't allow for retreating off the playing field and into the "comfort" of patienthood. Karl Von Durkheim (1971) illuminated the call to boldness as the difference between the two ways of relating:

> The man, who, being really on the Way, falls upon hard times in the world will not, as a consequence, turn to that friend who offers him refuge and comfort and encourages his old self to survive. Rather, he will seek out someone who will faithfully and inexorably help him to risk himself, so that he may endure the suffering and pass courageously through it. Only to the extent that man exposes himself over and over to annihilation, can that which is indestructible arise within him. In this lies the dignity of daring. (41–42)

The ensuing feedback from the world eventually leads us to a place in productive society where we thrive, where we're nurtured, where we contribute, and finally where we discover meaning and purpose in life.

THERE'S NO LID

After reading my material so far the well-intentioned therapist, psychologist, psychiatrist, friend, or family member may say: "Well that may work with some people, but he doesn't know ________ (a particular person considered "mentally ill")." "Or, we've tried that already. It may work for some but not ________?"

I'm here to tell you you don't know "________"! There is no set or fixed "________." You are not seeing them as they are! You're seeing him/her as you are. Even a consensus as to how _______ "is" doesn't prove anything as everyone uses (or in reality is used by) diagnostic or other totalizing labels (e.g., lazy, evil) and therefore suffers from a lack of interpersonal skill. You're seeing them as they've been conditioned! What you're seeing in front of you is someone whose identity, actions, feelings, beliefs, and thoughts have been, by virtue of the malleability of the human brain and human subjectivity, conditioned by those around him or her—past and present. The observer does in many ways powerfully effect (dare I say create) the observed. The "patient" is a social construction. Yes, society does construct so-called "mental illness." Recall from throughout prior chapters how our minds and identities are a product of our discursive relations. Subjectivity is intersubjectively constituted. We're created in relationship and communication with others. This book is here to argue that society can *deconstruct*, as well as construct, so-called "mental illness."

Moreover, whatever "you've tried" has been superficially layered on the rock bed of presuppositions, beliefs, and attitudes—not the least of which is the clinical worldview—that defeat your efforts, even if you try to hide these insidious and pervasive influences. Those of us familiar with subjectivity know that it can't be hidden; the body is broadcasting it ceaselessly and other bodies read it impeccably despite what's going on at the conscious level.

In 1976, the film *One Flew Over the Cuckoo's Nest* won five academy awards. In 1993, the film was deemed "culturally, historically, or aesthetically significant" by the United States Library of Congress. At the time the true significance of the film could not be recognized.

Indeed, "All the world's a stage, and all the men and women merely players."[2] In the mental health profession some people play the role of doctor, therapist, social worker, nurse, psychologist and other people play the role of patient. This is an existential perspective. To not understand the nature of social roles and instead to identify with them is to be at their effect, to be "hollow" (T. S. Eliot) and a "specialist without spirit" (Max Weber). It goes without saying that we can't dispense with roles, but we can gain cognitive distance from our roles and our roles can be informed by a vocabulary (such as is contained in this book) and commitment that give us greater connection, authenticity, compassion, openness, flexibility, subject-to-subject (adult-to-adult) relating, and respect for the dignity of the people we meet with. Moreover, we don't want to create roles, such as "the patient," that *defeat from the start* our efforts to empower another. With the right change in paradigm (read: vocabulary) "the patient" is transformed into the artist, the author, the intellectual, the musician, the poet.

NOTES

1. William Shakespeare, *Macbeth*, Act 5, Scene 5, 2.
2. William Shakespeare, *As You Like It*, Act 2, Scene 7, 139–66.

TEN

Unleash This Creativity onto the World

Creativity, imagination, passion, sensitivity, intelligence, and commitment are signal characteristics of people who have been relegated to the margins of society as the "mentally ill." The medicalization and pharmaceuticalization of the profession has had untold consequences in terms of wasted human capital. How many Virginia Wolfes, Friedrich Nietzsches, Charles Dickenses, Michelangelos, Winston Churchills, Ernest Hemingways, Isaac Newtons, Vincent Van Goghs, Tennessee Williamses, John Keatses, Leo Tolstoys, and Ludwig van Beethovens (to name a few) have instead been transformed into passive and insecure patients? What these people have in common is unparalleled creativity, imagination, sensitivity, intelligence, and originality that they employed to usher in new paradigms and eras of exploration and development. The so-called "mentally ill" contain within their ranks leaders of humanity.

If creative and imaginative people are at the margins of society, then who occupies the center? So-called "healthy," "normal" people? As it turns out we are all still struggling with adapting to the complexity of modernity. On the one hand, creative people identify with (and are therefore driven) by their feelings and have difficulty conforming; while on the other, so-called "normal" people are driven by conformity and identify more with their social roles. The "pathological" side of "normal" is also, in a sense, the highest performing: people embodying the Machiavellian identity. This is where deception and ruthlessness have become virtues—ends justifying means—à la Niccolo Machiavelli. This identity abounds in the corporate and political worlds.

One historical thread that has led to these rough classifications of human beings started during the Enlightenment. According to Norbert Elias (1978) in his book *The Civilizing Process: A History of Manners* medieval people were largely driven by their feelings and impulses. What we would call today moody, impulsive, violent, vulgar, and otherwise anti-social was the norm then (as it was in pre-Christian days). It wasn't until the sixteenth and seventeenth century, when French kings consolidated state power by shepherding the landed nobility into the French court at Versailles, that social norms tightened into criteria which (along with noble privilege) were to define membership in what was called *society*. The threshold at which a behavior was seen as embarrassing became lower and lower.

Instead of outright warfare, the French nobility in their "gilded cage" competed through an outward display of decorum, deference, and obsequiousness toward the established social hierarchy—combined with behind-the-scenes intrigue, deception, and ruthlessness—and vied for power and influence. Civility meant in those days how well one deferred to the established hierarchy; in one's station there were acceptable ways to treat those above and those below. Beneath this surface deference were the calculations of "stepping on necks" to move up the social stratum.

The French court was the center of Enlightenment civilization, later the middle class joined in the pretentious fray. The end result was a society based on what we could call a Machiavellian identity, where the ends justify the means and the pretense of civility hides ruthlessness, deception, and endless machinations.

One early critic of this early society based on ruthlessness, inauthenticity, and hypocrisy was Jean-Jacques Rousseau. Rousseau claimed that society corrupted what was otherwise a noble savage human being and that underneath the pretense and role-playing was an authentic self.

Rousseau was one of the fathers of the later period called romanticism which further emphasized feeling, sensitivity, imagination, unconventionality, and creativity. In *The Confessions* he demonstrated the legitimacy of the subjective. Nick Mansfield in his book *Subjectivity: Theories of the Self from Freud to Haraway* (2000) described Rousseau's breakthrough:

> Rousseau's achievement was to imagine the individual in total terms, to conceive of subjectivity in all its manifestations as a whole—not always consistent, not always admirable, not always logical, but at all times worthy of study and description. The sheer scale and intensity of individual experience entitles it to be the basis, starting-point and ground of all meaning. (20)

The romantics, in turn, profoundly influenced the eighteenth and nineteenth-century Russian authors who explored the vast unknown of the human inner experience, which later formed the foundation of psychological realism in literature, especially in the form of the novel.

While the Russian writers were depicting human *subjectivity*, the existentialists were exploring the place of the passions, commitment, choice, responsibility, freedom, authenticity, and leveraging our personal strengths in our engagement in the world. In short, the existentialists utilized passion, vision, and commitment in the service of human self-transcendence. The closest we could get to authenticity was to identify with our passions and commitments.

Figuratively speaking, as descendants of Rousseau (the lineage including the romanticists, the existentialists, the artists, the intellectuals, the poets, the literati) with feeling, creativity, sensitivity, and imagination as our greatest assets—with the right perspective and language—we can transform unwieldy feeling, imagination, and sensitivity into passion, commitment, and vision in such a way as to not only find a contributing place in productive society, but in transforming that very society for the better.

As we will see in the next section what is a liability (or deficit) in the medicalized context is an asset (or strength) in the larger humanistic and, in many cases, commercial context. Richard Florida in his book *The Rise of the Creative Class—Revisited* (2012) identifies the new societal demand for creativity and imagination:

> The Creative Class has the power, talent, and numbers to play a big role in reshaping our world. Its members—in fact, all of society—now have the opportunity to turn their introspection and soul searching into real energy for broader renewal and transformation. (loc. 358)

However, since our institutions as they currently exist demand conformity, integrating the creative class will likely be a creative challenge itself.

Another natural arena for creative people to contribute, for those inclined, would be activism in the mental health arena, helping to implement the perspective brought forth in this book, among other things.

So we have, roughly speaking, two strains of the post-Enlightenment secular identity. People who identify with their roles and people who identify with their feelings. Of course, in reality, there are vast and varied permutations of the way each of us relate to role and feeling, or reason and feeling. Moreover, role-identified people often go to psychotherapy to get in touch with their feelings. The problem for all of us is the integration of role (or reason) and feeling. Importantly, for our purposes we want to recognize how feeling-identified people are by and large unconventional and role-identified people are by and large conventional.

Furthermore, as we will see in chapter 11 people do not choose which they will identify with (or how these two tendencies will coalesce, combine, or compartmentalize), it's all a matter of happenstance, both in terms of genetic and early childhood conditioning. Identifying with roles has its obvious advantage in the workplace, whereas identifying with feelings serves us better in creative, imaginative, and otherwise artistic endeavors. One can begin to imagine how these two types work together: creative people forge new vistas of human exploration; conventional people institutionalize these new avenues for the benefit of all. But, as we saw in chapter 9, which world we inhabit—filled with patients or artists—depends on the words we use. Autistic is one letter and one paradigm away from artistic.

NO PERSONAL FAILING

One of the assumed benefits of the disease model was that people could explain their difficulties with the people and circumstances in their lives by ascribing those problems to their "illness." This is an understandable palliative. We all, for better or worse, have egos and comparisons are omnipresent. By nature we peck each other into order and arrange hierarchically. I once had a client who told me that he likes his psychiatric diagnosis because without it he would see himself as an "F'd-up person."

In order to address this issue I'm not going to further elevate mental health consumers, instead, I'm going to lower all the rest of us. In order to do so I need to provide some background.

The 2007 financial crisis was a watershed moment in history. Prior to the crisis the American stock market and financial institutions were largely held in esteem. There were blemishes to be sure, of which the Savings and Loan debacle and Enron scandal were emblematic. But, overall, the titans of the financial industry were highly regarded and perhaps even viewed as heroes and exemplars of the American dream and U.S. economy. In 2007, it was reported that 47 percent of Harvard graduates left Harvard to go to work at Wall Street (Zauzmer, 2013).

As the details of the crisis were revealed it became clear that many of the so-called "heroes" of the economy were in reality moral midgets. The greedy machinations and deceptions revealed deep flaws in character. People we looked up to turned out to be disdainfully corrupt. Though there is much more to tell, both good and bad, about the U.S. financial industry the point I'm making is that the 2007 crisis was a great disillusionment. The corruption on Wall Street reflected the moral bankruptcy of its inhabitants. Of course, the same can be said about our politicians, only the disillusionment started much earlier, around the time of Watergate.

Post-2007 we see a widening gap between the haves and have-nots, where the haves accumulate wealth with means that produce less value and employment than ever before in U.S. history. The evidence for corporate and political corruption amasses daily. So in other words, what were once leaders to be emulated are now pariahs to be tolerated.

In terms of disillusionment the 2007 crisis was akin to that of World War I (WWI). Prior to WWI the Western world was filled with the enthusiasm of the Enlightenment. Progress, toleration, capitalism, and reason seemed boundless in their ability to better humankind. However the incomprehensible horrors and death toll of WWI crushed this optimism. Western culture had confronted the leviathan of human irrationality beneath the thin film of reasonable and polite society, and it responded with Sigmund Freud's unconscious, surrealism, stream of consciousness, and psychological realism in literature. World War II furthered our unmooring from any kind of moral certainty.

Not to be too hard on the wealthy and powerful, I believe them to simply be the best at what so many of the rest of us also do (also, let's not forget that power corrupts). As I mentioned earlier in this chapter, the prevailing autonomy is Machiavellian. Our ability to hold down a job and maintain relationships has much to do with our ability to identify with roles and, to varying degrees, to employ the use of pretense and deception. From this perspective ends justify means and off our soul goes to market. A case could be made for the Machiavellian identity being a diagnostic category in its own right if we were to envision a new and better "normal."

So from this point of view the sensitive, imaginative, unconventional, and creative person just hasn't traversed that Machiavellian path. In terms of performing our functional roles, identifying with fickle feelings leaves us inconsistent at best and withdrawn from life at worst. But, so goes the life of the artist, the musician, the imaginative intellectual, the philosopher, the spiritual leader, and the writer. The difficulty adapting to roles is a liability in one setting, an asset in another. The mainspring of human creativity lies unbridled in feeling and imagination. Society nurtures creativity by refusing to pathologize and ostracize the unconventionality that comes with it. Unconventionality is the flip side of creativity.

One venue for creativity is business. The modern bureaucratized world demands that we take on roles and harmoniously fit into the mechanism of our institutions. Yes, Machiavelli has benefited us all. On the other hand, fortuitously, today's businesses are looking for imagination and creativity. Bruce Nussbaum et al. put it this way in *Bloomberg Business* (2005):

> The Knowledge Economy as we know it is being eclipsed by something new—call it the Creativity Economy. . . . Increasingly, the new core competence is creativity—the right brain stuff that smart companies are now harnessing to generate top-line growth. The game is changing. It isn't just about math and science anymore. It's about creativity, imagination, and, above all, innovation.

Bob Deutsch, a cognitive anthropologist writing for the *Huffington Post* (2013), equates creativity with competitiveness and puts a new spin on so-called "manic episodes":

> Creativity and innovation are critical to any business enterprise if it is going to thrive in our fast-changing world and craft a future of ex-

> panded opportunity. In this complex and volatile business context, everyone—a Fortune 100 CEO with a long tenure, a newly minted serial entrepreneur, as well as each and every corporate employee—needs to become a "corporate creative." . . . Creativity requires being attuned to your own experience from moment-to-moment. A creative person lives life on an emotional roller-coaster, and likes it that way. Creatives tolerate the dips because they want the stimulation on the upswing. Creatives live in feeling because that's where the revelatory cues are that spark innovation.

But the corporate world, which is typically founded on conformity and convention, needs to adapt in such a way as to integrate these unwieldy, non-conventional, and creative folks. At the same time, creative people need training in fitting into the institutional grid by sourcing their greatest passion, the commitment to the quality of their lives. From this big-picture perspective our long-term freedom and prosperity depends in many ways on our ability to play by the rules.

Whether the creative class chooses to join the institutional world or express their creativity in a less confining atmosphere, the imperative is the same: society needs to make room for creativity and creative people and to do this we need to get rid of the pathologizing, thus marginalizing, vocabulary. The only "condition" anyone suffers from is the *human condition*. On the other hand, since our institutions as they are presently constituted demand conformity, integrating the creative class is likely to be a creative challenge in itself.

Clients, as exemplified by the one mentioned in the beginning of this chapter, often see themselves through the normative/conventional lens of the prevailing conceptual reality. This is an example of how one can participate in one's own subjugation without really knowing it. They have accepted society's normative/conventional definition of them (e.g., some version of being an F'd-up person). The psychiatric label serves as a mitigating factor (an "illness" explains their difficulties) which makes them more acceptable to themselves and to others; but only so within the prevailing normative/conventional reality. From the larger context we can live with their unconventional ways in order to benefit from their genius. The client mentioned at the beginning was a highly sought after consultant in the video gaming industry.

As I will mentioned in the postmodern narrative chapter (11), the best neuroscience to date and the greatest philosophical minds of the twentieth century tell us that none of us have authored ourselves, as the Apostle Paul said, "Everything you have is received." From this "spiritual" perspective no one deserves any applause, nor anyone any scorn—judgment disappears. We're all "thrown" into the world only to wake up to find what cards we've been dealt. When will we recognize our fundamental sameness—that we're all in the same boat? Far from the cliché, this is a recognition that will profoundly change your life.

AN IMPORTANT NOTE TO FAMILY AND FRIENDS

We're all—client, therapist, psychiatrist, mom, dad, brother, sister, neighbor, husband, friend, wife, etc.—in the same predicament of subjectivity. We're all on the path of human transformation. We all suffer from the same condition, *the human condition*. We're all in the same boat. To identify someone in your life as "the problem" (a "patient" or a person who's "mentally ill") is to see yourself as "a victim" and to consequently retreat from the playing field of life and relationships. "Victimhood" is very, very contagious. The negotiation of rules of conduct, fairness, the exchange of points of view, the resolution of conflict, mutual respect, and the exchange of equivalent value is a perennial problem on the playing field of human relationships. Review chapter 6 on the effect of labels on relationships.

When someone in your life is behaving in a manner that is destructive toward themselves, you, or the relationship then this amounts to a practical problem of the social world. We need to posit a "mental illness" as much as we need to posit "evil spirits." And the more you care about them, the more important is this truth. Care too often becomes control. Interdependence becomes co-dependence. Moreover, care is often comingled with judgmentalness.

Recall from our earlier discussion that the judgmental mind owns us if we're not careful. Judging people is what we call in the postmodern world cultural agency. By way of family, peers, media, or any other kind of social grouping we become simply agents or representatives of culture's dictates, prejudices, ways of living, normatives, and values—we're meme machines. None of us have carefully thought through and concluded these values, etc.; we simply "know what's right and know what's wrong"—certainty is the defining characteristic of our subjugation. Or we might rebel against the status quo, with the same rigidity and certainty only in the opposite direction. Or our enculturation could be laissez-faire to the point of indifference—still we feel certain this attitude is right!

The point is that people with unconventional—sometimes uncooperative, eccentric, counterproductive, impulsive, rebellious, imaginative, slothful, unfair, creative, or even destructive—behavior are subject to the force of judgment (the "gaze" would be included here) and labeling by the significant "other." What we're left with is the battle of wills. When it's about being "more normal" then the person's only two options are to submit or rebel. Submitting is often a Pyrrhic victory where the battle is won at the cost of the war. This is, in effect, delayed parenting done to adults.

For example, the culture loves to identify and punish "laziness." Remember that our subjectivity determines our being. A person watching TV all night and sleeping all day is acting perfectly in accord with his or her subjectivity. From his/her frame of reference this slothful living makes perfect sense—likely indicating a deep sense of helplessness, hopelessness, or resignation. This is true despite their conscious (surface) recognition that they should be being more productive. Real and lasting behavior change involves alteration in subjectivity, or what we postmodernists would call resubjectification. This is why the unpacking of subjectivity and the exploration of intersubjectivity are the main events in postmodern coaching.

The answer to this dilemma, short of getting involved in postmodern coaching or the like, is simple but difficult: respect the person's choices and help them get what they want while enforcing your boundaries and limitations. So rather than being directive and judgmental about getting with the cultural program (i.e., enforcing what you think this person "should do"), we privilege a person's decisions and support them in getting what they want by offering various perspectives and recommended courses of action through persuasion and inspiration. Of course, this is very simplified and other factors certainly come into play (e.g., our persuasive efforts often amount to power struggles). Moreover, in relationships we have limitations and boundaries in terms of resources, time, etc.; and like all human relationships considerations of fairness come into play. So for example, in the paragraph above where the "person" is an adult "son" living with his parents, the parents have every right (indeed are obligated) to demand that he be productive (get a job or go to school) in exchange for room and board. The key is *how* this is done.

Another factor to keep in mind is that people are often ambivalent about behavior change and/or taking steps toward achieving their objectives. This means that one day a person may be excited and motivated about getting a job, but the next day have an aversion to doing so when insecurity arises when the prospect of rejection or failure looms, or in his/her mind independence might be equated with alienation. When people are ambivalent our persuasive efforts can result in the other person digging in their heels—resistance is co-created. To get an appreciation for ambivalence, stages of change, and how we co-create resistance or co-create motivation I recommend William Miller and Stephen Rollnick's (2002) classic *Motivational Interviewing*.

Then there's the issue of fluctuating motivation. Remember Shakespeare: "What to ourselves in passion we propose, / The passion ending, doth the purpose lose."[1] In other words, passions are fickle, they come and go, and with them so goes our motivation and goal-directed behavior. All projects have their honeymoon phase. A week or month later we may have even forgotten about what we were so excited about. Over time, with better languaging and practice identifying with our commitment, we get better at being responsible for maintaining our engagement, motivation, and momentum.

If we understand the truth of human subjectivity that people are all doing the best they can given the resources (mind, body, circumstances, etc.) they have, then our relationship problems become about behavior. The problem is in our current medication-centered universe behavior problems are always languaged in terms of "illness" with "medications" as the cure. When all you have is a hammer, everything looks like a nail. A typical example of this is when a parent insists that their son or daughter "take their medication" because when they don't all hell breaks loose. What the mother or father really wants is behavior change and they think the only means is "medications."

Let's examine what's really going on when someone insists that "the other take their medications." Recall there's a content and command aspect to every communication. The content (or denotation) is more or less the assertion: I recommend you take your medications because you have a "chemical imbalance" and I think that would help you with your behavior, which, by the way, is a problem for me. The command (or connotative) aspect is: I'm normal, you're not, so you should listen to me. You're a patient and you're not responsible for your behavior, your behavior is a function of whether or not the chemicals in your brain are in balance or not; but what you *are* responsible for is "taking your medications." Furthermore, whatever *my* part in your behavior is is negligible compared to your "imbalance." This completely disregards and invalidates the person's (client's) subjective framework and all the contextual variables that go into a person's perceptions, feelings, and actions. If they simply *comply* they do so at the cost of their long-term self-responsibility. The beloved idea of *compliance* is the ultimate irony. Another battle won at the cost of the war.

Having said all this, the most respectful way to deal with counterproductive behavior is to deal with the behavior. Learn to set firm limits, ultimatums if necessary—and stick to them. In effect, what you're saying is "I don't care how you do it; but the behavior's got to change." Given the stress and pressure of the demand (the credibility of which is gained through consistency and follow-through) one might consider all options, including pills. Now you're positioning the person as responsible and we can assign the beloved question "Have you taken your medications?" to the category of being just one more misguided attempt at *fixing* someone. Ask Co-Dependents Anonymous (the experts in this area) if fixing someone is a good idea. Care has to be balanced with respect; respect for the other as a responsible adult.

When I talk with friends and family about these and other strategies, I sometimes get the response "We've already tried that." Well, the truth is you haven't already tried that. Or if you've tried it you've tried it from your already existing mindset or subjective framework—which means you're just doing more of the same expecting different results. Just one more example of how important the quality of our subjectivity is to the quality of our relationships.

In summary, a simple formula for empowerment is as follows. Be person-centered. Listen and take the other seriously. Allow for them to choose their means as well as their ends. Know that people are motivated for something, even if it's to find something to be motivated about. The rule is to only provide those tools that will help your loved one get what they want. Secondly, know where the reasonable limits and boundaries are; set them and be consistent, especially when living together. When it comes to limits, insist on ends (usually behavior change), not means. Thirdly, allow for ambivalence; change has stages and it's unrealistic to expect people be consistent in their motivation, initiative, and action. Fourthly, recognize and appreciate incremental progress. Finally, know that life experience is a much better teacher than well-intended instruction and advice. Be OK with however your loved one chooses. There is no failure, only information.

And most of all, I highly recommend that all concerned become conversant in this vocabulary of empowerment (e.g., postmodern coaching) in order to get and keep the right perspective. Attitude is everything, and attitude is wholly a function of perspective.

NOTE

1. William Shakespeare, *Hamlet*, Act 3, Scene 2.

ELEVEN

A Postmodern Narrative—the Subjectivity of Compassion

We've talked a lot about therapist authenticity with respect to empathy and unconditional positive regard as essential to the healing relational stance necessary for attunement, alliance, and intersubjectivity. The coalescence of these qualities is not something that can be willed out of nothing, intuited, nor does it occur naturally with little or no effort (e.g., wisdom that comes with age), nor is it taught in graduate school, nor can it be pretended, nor is it the result of some privileged access to some absolute or metaphysical reality (à la Plato). It is a particular multidisciplinary vantage point acquired from experience, education, and transformation. This book is part of that vantage point. Freedom from the judgmental mind is a lifelong endeavor, but well worthwhile. Below is an example of a postmodern narrative that recognizes our common human subjective dilemma and as a consequence supports an experience of humility and compassion.

I'm aware that postmodernists abhor grand or universal narratives, but without them we're left with relativism, moral relativism included. To contradict Friedrich Nietzsche from a particular practical point of view, there are some things we have to call "facts." Though not absolute, the word "fact" is still a useful term of art. For example, in this book we call neuroplasticity fact and "chemical imbalances" fiction. We do so out of both a correspondence with our observation of nature (i.e., mapping nature) as well as employing utility as criteria for truth and for use of language, metaphor, and interpretation. Furthermore, there is an interplay between the correspondence view of reality and the linguistic view of reality. Like Martin Heidegger asserts, "Words, like the chisel of the carver, can create what never existed before rather than simply describe what already exists." In other words, words do describe or represent things that exist; we say this in order to stay grounded in the practical and material world. Correspondence with the physical world of things (i.e., "mapping nature") is a point of view to be judged according to *its* utility. Whether we're talking about the creational or representational use of language, there are certain things we can say are "facts" because of their consistency, evidence, and utility. I say all this to say that in this chapter and throughout the book we do establish certain context-dependent facts then use language to better interpret those "facts" all with an eye toward usefulness.

Human beings comprehend existence in terms of stories or narratives. During the late eighteenth century Immanuel Kant (and later the twentieth-century cognitive scientists) claimed that the categories of such comprehension—space, time, causality, substance, etc.—are imposed on the world by the human brain. Space, time, and causality coalesce into narrative. In short, we all have a life story.

Our life story acts as a context from which we interpret ourselves and our circumstances. Our subjective take on any given person or situation is embedded in our life story—a life story largely defined in early childhood by the significant others in our lives. Hence, without knowing it, because we interpret people and situations consistently in terms of our life story, in a self-fulfilling manner, we are destined to repeat our story throughout our lives—same story, different actors.

Part of the reason it happens like this is that the incredibly adaptable and malleable brain of the child becomes patterned and more or less fixed in terms of a personality by about age six. Christopher Nave in his 2010 paper "On the Contextual Independence of Personality"—published in six journals on almost as many continents—provided convincing evidence that personality (character) is formed by age six and is remarkably stable throughout adulthood. Yet, researchers tell us the foundation for the personality is set by age three.

The developing brain starts off with amazing flexibility and range of receptiveness and responsiveness; with increasing age and experience it, in a sense, commits to the environment in which it finds itself by "hard-wiring" the neuronal circuits—through myelination and synaptic pruning—in such a way that they operate far more quickly and efficiently. What the brain gains in efficiency it loses in flexibility. As a result neuroplasticity declines precipitously from age zero to three years (Huttenlocher, 1979). By age three the way a child has been conditioned to *emotionally react* to the world is formed and set. It does this to increase the speed of response. By age six further pruning and myelination—in response to further social conditioning—results in a more differentiated albeit more patterned set of responses we call a personality.

Apparently, at least in terms of our ancestral environments (presumably far more consistent throughout the entire life span than today), the payoff in speed was worth the cost in terms of flexibility. This timeline of human brain development would account for all the emphasis and resource in recent years applied to early intervention educational and developmental programs for ages zero to five (Allen and Duncan Smith, 2010).

Though the personality is fixed by age six, the brain's higher neocortical functions continue their malleability much later, into a person's mid-twenties (Siegel, 2014). The higher level, neocortical, areas increase their reorganizing capacity as the lower (emotional) areas decrease their flexibility. So from age three onward with continued language acquisition the child begins to *narratively interpret* the world. However, because the emotional base is fixed at age three and the personality is fixed at age six the range of interpretation is increasingly narrowed. Though we may choose how high a house may be, how many windows and rooms, what kind of carpet or floors to use, etc., the foundation set in the beginning limits and in many ways determines all of what's subsequently possible.

So by age six the human brain is effectively fixed in such a way that absent a program later in life to facilitate neuronal change we live out our lives on autopilot. As the ancient Greeks put it: character is destiny. Or, as T. S. Eliot (1970) declared, "In my beginning is my end." Once again because of our theoretical ontology (seeing the world through the categories of science and social discourse versus experience) we had to wait for neuroscience to tell us what was obvious to the pre-moderns and those poets among us today—we had to wait 2,500 years for science to confirm what was easily perceived by the ancients.

What this tells us is not only is there a consistency of character throughout a lifetime, but that that character determines our life-world. We just keep repeating our default narrative in different situations and with different people. When it comes to character, any neuroplasticity we see in adulthood varies in the degree that we're able to intervene on long-standing patterns of being.

This brings up questions of choice and free will. Many neuroscientists and critical philosophers have concluded that free will and choice are largely illusory. What looks like a choice is really the brain commenting on an action which was unconsciously "decided" milliseconds before it was consciously "decided" and then performed (Libet et al., 1982). Our "conscious decisions" are little more than an afterthought. Benjamin Libet claimed that at best we have veto power over our brain's unconscious decisions; in other words, we do possess "free won't."

Twentieth-century philosophers and literary critics complicated the matter of free will even further with two contrasting views. The existentialists understood human beings as self-determining and capable of making responsible choices. The structuralists, the successors of the existentialists, claimed that there are cultural and linguistic structures that construct our identities (subjectivity) and limit what can be thought, and consequently limit our freedom and choice. The postmodernists did away with binaries and claimed that both are true. In other words, to the extent that we can recognize and transcend the impress of culture and nature as they manifest in us we can choose outside of the available cultural and natural options of thought and action.

For our purposes we don't need to settle the question of free will and choice, we can simply assume that when considering the major determinant of our behavior, our personality, we may have far less free will and choice than we think. I believe this insight to be constitutive of our recognition of subjectivity as the replacement for the idea of an inner self. Subjectivity has long been the subject of the postmodernists. Personality is a manifestation of patterned subjectivity.

Now let's get back to the narrative that was imprinted on us by others. When people impose their will on children (aka parenting) they are actually acting as agents of culture actively defining and judging the child's self, actions, emotions, and world in terms of the available cultural definitions. The act of "judging" right/wrong, good/bad, beautiful/ugly occurs automatically and often with great force (thus the recipient's experience of shame, humiliation, ridicule, embarrassment, etc.). This is the manner in which cultural values and practices are transmitted from generation to generation. This process happens with so little conscious deliberation as to prompt some philosophers to propose that ideas or memes (defined as the basic unit of culture) use our bodies as hosts in their continual battle to prevail and reproduce. Though memetics most likely represents an exaggeration, it does highlight the extent to which we unwarily and involuntarily represent the culture which was imposed on us. Or, as Nietzsche put it, the will to power is expressed by the need to impose values and ways of living on "the other." The judgmental mind is culture's blind press.

The culture, in turn, is historically determined. Human culture evolves. But at any given time the prevailing cultural values and practices (i.e., discourses) are thrust upon the developing child and eventually becomes his/her narratively constituted worldview or subjectivity. There's no escaping how each of us is a product of history in its current expression we call culture.

However, the problem lies in the fact that we are standing on a culturally and linguistically constituted vantage point and don't realize it. Like water is to the fish, the world as it appears to us seems like objective reality.

Putting all this together, by the time we're age six we have a brain that is patterned—by virtue of genetics and childhood conditioning—to interpret the rest of our lives inflexibly in terms of our childhood experience, which was defined by people who could largely only represent cultural discourse; parenting is enculturating. We're on autopilot.

Even as an adult when we begin to base our decisions on our adult experience, how we comprehend that experience and the very ability to learn from that experience was implanted by nature and nurture before we were even aware of ourselves.

How this plays out day to day, moment by moment is a follows. Every moment of our existence our actions are perfectly in accord with the way in which the world is showing up. Interpretation and response are a unity, just different aspects of the same phenomenon. The "showing up" is embedded in a life story composed prior to age six. So from this very broad and deep point of view every human being is doing the best they can given what they have to work with. Furthermore, in order to change our actions we need to change the way in which the world shows up which also involves altering the narrative that supports this "showing up."

Moreover, our subjectivity based in our default narrative, like writ large in the mental health system, is self-enclosed and self-affirming, making it practically impossible to incorporate experience which contradicts it. This explains why people often learn very slowly or not at all from experience.

So this is the state of the early twenty-first-century peopled world in which we live. *We know not what we do.*[1] From this compassionate point of view we can stop judging others and see, perhaps for the first time, the playing field of life. The world and its human inhabitants are neither positive nor negative. No bad people, no good people; no bad behavior, no good behavior. As Shakespeare and the ancient Stoics agreed: "There is nothing either good or bad but thinking makes it so."[2] It's just behavior; behavior we encounter on the playing field of life. Our victim-like experience (as seen through the lens of our childhood narrative; no surprise!) is really a cause and consequence of a lack of perspective and practice-dependent skill on the playing field of life.

At six weeks old, Adolf Hitler was a cute little baby. The people in his life inculcated him with the cultural conditions (including ideologies) at the time thus shaping the historical figure we're familiar with. Even with due consideration to biological substrate, our minds and personalities are to a large degree socially constructed. Social discourses (i.e., social values and practices) are embodied in each of us. Though as our "mind" we experience them very personally and privately, it doesn't change the fact that we absorbed them from the outside, from our communications with others. We represent these discourses. To the extent that we *lack* "socialization" (good, bad, or otherwise) we are subject to our natural instincts. Though mammals and primates show affinitive instincts, they're largely dominated by indifferent and antagonistic instincts. The male grizzly bear will kill its own offspring for food and in order to have sexual access to the mother. Hierarchies and reproductive rights are brutally established with no regard to fairness or justice. We too have the predatory and sexual instincts of our animal relatives.

When we mix ideologies (which reference the absolute) with the will to power (animal antagonism and rivalry) we can get genocide. The power of language and ideology is a double-edged sword as it can be used to resonate with either our antagonistic or affinitive instincts, and how this happens in each of us individually depends on the happenstance of the time and place of our birth. Humanity is in conflict with itself—the post-modern worldview being a step in the resolution of this conflict.

As tempting as it is to give credit to people for their achievements or judge those for their lack thereof, from a neuroscience point of view no one gets credit—not even "good" parents. This is because the foundation for all our learning and choices was set practically before we even became aware of ourselves. This is true even for our capacity to learn. So whether we're talking about Mother Teresa or Osama Bin Ladin, the president of the United States or an out of control homeless person, Steve Jobs or those who perpetrate internet fraud (and I don't mean to imply value judgments by the comparisons) neither gets credit or criticized—in both cases their genetics, early childhood conditioning, and circumstantial advantages/disadvantages determined their choices, possibilities, and destinies—in both cases, neither is self-authored. The Apostle Paul had it right when he declared:

> For who maketh thee to differ from another? and what hast thou that thou didst not receive? Now if thou didst receive it, why dost thou glory, as if thou hadst not received it?[3]

Even if we had the capacity to be original that too would have been determined before age six. The idea that there is a self inside us making good or bad choices is the great myth of Cartesius (René Descartes's Latin name).

Of course, social and religious institutions rely on the idea of free will and the idea that a person could have chosen otherwise; this is the basis for punishment and damnation, respectively. Again, how receptive we are to laws and religious doctrine as well as to learning from consequences are a function of our pre-determined personality.

So where does this leave us? It leaves us in a very humble place, subject to subject, where no one is any better than anyone else. We're all in the same boat called unaddressed and transparent subjectivity. At the very least this should infuse a big dose of humility and compassion into ourselves and our relationships.

Civilization is a developmental process. During the Middle Ages we resembled beasts much more than we do now. Mood swings, impulsive or antisocial behavior were the norm in pre-modern societies (Elias, 1978). Going further back, in the days before Christianity, you might describe us as without conscience, and back then it was probably a good thing! As my favorite historians Will and Arial Durant used to say, "Yesterday's virtues are today's vices." Moreover, ontogeny recapitulates phylogeny; in other words, we can observe all these historical stages recapitulated in child development (Gould, 1977; Spock, 1968, 229; Freud, 1950; Piaget, 1933).

So people displaying mood swings or impulsive or antisocial behavior simply didn't have the historically generated, culturally/linguistically transmitted training. They don't *have* "borderline personality disorders" or "antisocial personality disorders"; they're just being anachronistic, displaying appropriate responses, only in the wrong historical epoch!

So vocabularically realized human subjectivity is the answer to our animal instincts. It has developed over time and its best aspects are not equally distributed. Not all of us get exposed to the best part of humanity's subjectivity and therefore we do the best we can. Without sufficient training (e.g., parenting or coaching) people can act in ways that are counterproductive or harmful to other people. Even intentionally harmful, vengeful, vindictive, even homicidal behavior reflects nature's raw antagonism coalesced with ego or ideology. In other words, what we might otherwise call "evil" is far from self-authored. Neither is its opposite, "good"; the "good" people of the world are in every way equally on autopilot. Whether one is "good" or "bad" is solely determined by the happenstance of genetics and time and place of birth, none of which was of our own choosing. All is received. We know not what we do.

A better word for bad behavior is natural behavior, that is, due to a lack of training we're run by our predatory or otherwise antagonistic instincts.

This postmodern narrative is being expressed by many in one form or another. Its tenets can be found in historical, literary, scientific, philosophical, or religious texts as well as in spirituality or self-help literature. One of the effects of this narrative should be to greatly mitigate the self- and other-antagonism (including judgmentalness) and the ubiquitous hierarchical comparisons that cloud our path to personal responsibility and compassion through the medium of language.

A NOTE ABOUT PERSONAL RESPONSIBILITY AND SOCIAL VALUE

Having said all of the above, I don't mean to imply that there is no such thing as personal responsibility or social value. I'm just saying that personal responsibility is available to all of us to varying degrees and its access, for starters, varies depending on factors that we had nothing to do with. To intervene on our genetic and socially conditioned destiny is a monumental effort, and most of us with some significant effort merely steer our lives within their confines. We can decide to live in Miami or Chicago, go to this or that school, take up skiing, "reinvent ourselves," and on and on. I'm just saying that personal responsibility is an ever-evolving ideal of civilization whose access is dependent on our spiritual transformation which, in turn, is dependent on addressing human subjectivity.

Furthermore, there's no question that those who produce value to humanity are in a sense more valuable to humanity. Moreover, there's no question humanity has self-destructive tendencies of which some of us are representative. My point is none of us *chose* where we stand vis-à-vis humanity's struggle with itself.

In summary, whether we realize it or not, we're all on the path of spiritual/personal growth. The idea that some of us are "normal" and on the path of spiritual/personal growth while others have mental disorders and are in need of "treatment" is a complete fabrication. We're all equal in the realm of human transformation and all equally challenged by human subjectivity. Moreover, more material success or social skill is a result of (1) an autopilot (or personality) set in early childhood through circumstance and genetics that were favorable in these areas and (2) patterns of being which themselves could be classified as abnormal (i.e., the Machiavellian identity). Creativity, imagination, sensitivity, intelligence, vision, and originality are likewise "received."

So it is from this vantage point that the Rogerian conditions—unconditional positive regard, accurate empathy, and therapist congruence (or authenticity)—fall into alignment and the gateway to compassion and intersubjectivity are opened.

NOTES

1. Bible, King James Version, Luke 23:34.
2. William Shakespeare, *Hamlet* Act 2, scene 2, 239–51.
3. Bible, King James Version, 1 Corinthians 4:7.

IV

The Art Form

TWELVE

The New Psychology Is an Art Form

Around the time of the Renaissance, science began to usurp the search for truth from its progenitor, philosophy. In the modern era, science became increasingly specialized, giving rise to, among others, the social sciences. Not surprisingly the social sciences would also stake claim to truth in their respective domains. However, as we've discovered so far in this book social sciences (including psychology and psychiatry) have a very tenuous connection to science, namely in statistical studies; however the labels and concepts based on statistical studies represent a particular point of view, interpretation, and vocabulary, not scientific truth, nor do they "map nature." Moreover, thanks to Immanuel Kant and Friedrich Nietzsche in particular, we recognize that the human brain is incapable of access to absolute truth, but instead is an organ of adaptation whose main tool is language and metaphor. The human brain makes distinctions in language in order to help it deal with itself and its environment. Truth becomes about utility. Here's an example.

I once had a client who had just started a new job. His first impression was that his new employer was disorganized, inefficient, and overall incompetent. This initial description caused him great frustration, disappointment, and angst at having turned down other attractive job offers. As I created the space for his subjectivity to unfold we realized that his fear of not having control over his circumstances and his unrealistic expectations were getting the best of him. At the instant of that recognition I blurted out, "You don't like puzzles!" He was surprised and a little stunned at the force of my pronouncement. He said, "As a matter of fact I love puzzles!" Problem solved.

The "puzzle" metaphor was not any sort of objective "truth," it was a metaphor that redescribed his situation such that he stopped resisting his work situation as it was, or said another way more generally, resisting life as it is. By immersing myself in his subjectivity the perfect redescription—as defined by its resonance and utility—exploded into the dialogue. The temporary coalescence of our subjectivities (intersubjectivity) brought forth the appropriate and timely aspect of human wisdom: that we're far better off not resisting life *as it is* while we're in the process of making it better. Our premature judgments can defeat us. Now he was in a much better position to learn new skills in suspending judgment and frustration while more open-mindedly and flexibly responding to the challenges that presented themselves.

We are moving from truth to metaphor, to a kind of poetry in service of rationality, constructive action, and subjective fulfillment. We should be addressing *being* itself rather than trying to prove it. Moreover, it is in the subject-to-subject intimacy that we *unconceal*—with attention, sensitivity, intention, language, and metaphor—either that which our client already knows or is ready to know. This is the art of psychotherapy. The master therapist is like Martin Heidegger's "true cabinet maker":

> In his discussion of thinking, Heidegger uses the analogy of a cabinetmaker's apprentice. In Heidegger's view this apprentice is not working on cabinets just for practice. He is not working merely in order to learn the trade. Learning the trade may bring these secondary results, but they are not primary reasons. The "true cabinetmaker," in his view, both answers and responds to different kinds of wood and to the shapes slumbering within the wood. (Krell 1993, 379) This example stands as an effective illumination of how poetry uncovers. The world and beings in the world are like wood freshly hewn from a burled tree. Each piece requires a different response in order to bring out its best characteristics. If the aspiring cabinetmaker were to treat each piece exactly the same he could probably create functional pieces at the cost of sacrificing much of the wood's beauty or power. The unique shapes "slumbering" in the wood require *Dasein's* interaction instead of mere "work" from the outside. "Uncovering" requires the cabinetmaker to go into the wood, to let it be by highlighting its peculiarities instead of cutting through them. Without that "relatedness" to the wood "the craft will never be anything but empty busywork." (Krell 1993, 379). A piece of wood, treated by a sensitive cabinetmaker, is uncovered in a very full sense. (Rogers, 2006)

Through our finely honed sensitivity and receptivity we see the "shapes slumbering within" our clients. Each client "requiring a different response in order to bring out its best characteristics." The unconcealing of the "shapes slumbering within" requires "interaction"; the therapist must "go into" the client, to let him or her be "by highlighting peculiarities rather than cutting through them." It is through such intersubjective "relatedness" that our clients are "uncovered in a very full sense."

On the other hand, "cutting through" the "peculiarities" in favor of similarities to be made into categories we instead "see" psychiatric diagnoses, "mental illness," symptoms (deficiencies), and are propelled into motion by the roles comprised by "assessment," "treatment," "case management," "testing," "needs assessment"; we are all but completely blind and unresponsive to the strengths, interests, preferences, needs, resourcefulness, concerns, insecurities, joys, temperament, language, values, and priorities, all of which constitutes the raw material for our art form.

The breakthrough that psychotherapy is an art form has been emerging in fits and starts for decades. The manualization of psychotherapy in the 1980s and 1990s was an attempt to shift focus from theory to practice, and in the process—especially with the employment of transcribed sessions that were analyzed and interpreted in detail—turned our attention to the in-the-moment subtleties of language, dialogue, and relationship. Indeed, master therapists have long recognized themselves as artists. James Bugental in his *The Art of the Psychotherapist: How to Develop the Skills That Take Psychotherapy beyond Science* (1987) asserts:

> Our fundamental assumptions have been that the most mature psychotherapists are more artists than technicians and that they bring to bear a wide variety of sensitivities and skills so their clients can release their latent potentials for fuller living. . . . The point is this: The dimensions in this book are not used in just these forms by master therapists. As I have set them out their chief function is to lead maturing therapists to such *further perceptions as will foster their developing their own further potentials*. (264–65; my italics added)

Yes, "further perceptions as will foster their developing their own further potentials"—psychotherapy as an art, like other arts, is about *perspective*. This includes the multidisciplinary (history, neuroscience, physics, literature, philosophy, biology, culture, epigenetics, etc.) perspective of this book which justifies and describes psychotherapy as an art form. And the practices are recursively related to the perspectives, each forever evolving through mutual influence. This contrasts with psychotherapy as a science where reductive truths (oversimplifications where a perspective on the whole is mistaken for the whole) and reified labels make psychotherapy rigid, formulaic, and unresponsive to the client.

As bold as this may seem, I'm redefining master therapist as *competent therapist*. All professional therapists should have the competence of an Irving Yalom, Carl Rogers, Carl Whitaker, Albert Ellis, Insoo Kim Berg, Scott Miller, Virginia Satir, Michael White, etc. This is a profound "raising of the bar" as far as competency goes. Yes, we're definitely raising the bar as far as competency goes, but with the right selection, education, and training this may not be as unrealistic as it sounds, in fact, this is already happening, albeit at a snail's pace.

The human brain is an organ of adaptation and as such despite the disabling effect of its language system, psychology has made incremental progress. In other words, therapists committed to *results* have learned effective techniques despite the gravitational pull of their categories and theories. Moreover, psychotherapy outcome research, interpersonal neurobiology, and postmodern theory and practice continue to point to the efficacy of relationship, engagement, mindfulness, attunement, nonjudgmental awareness, authenticity, and working within the client's frame of reference—all of which hinge on the therapist's subjectivity and dialogic skill. Furthermore, with a post–healthcare reform emphasis on outcomes, efficiency, prevention, and wellness there is greater and greater emphasis on what works versus a loyalty to old categories and theories.

What this boils down to is the recognition of psychotherapy and psychiatry as art forms. Helping modalities are expressions of co-creativity; they depend on the *moment-to-moment* listening and responding. The response to one statement or question informs the next. You can't have an inner monologue/commentary going on at the same time like the characters in some of Woody Allen's earlier movies.

This is a deep space of curiosity, uncertainty, and unknowing. It is a collaborative venture where both client and therapist enter into the same subjective space. This is in contrast to the typical way in which therapists have labels, categories, theories, and formulas with which to see (i.e., seemingly objectively assess), interpret, and "intervene" with the client. *Believing* the categories ("symptoms," "diagnoses," and other deficit language and clinical jargon) is *seeing* the categories to the exclusion of the nuances and subtleties of the client's inner world, its outer expressions, and its moment-to-moment changeability. Categories are crippling. Bugental (1987) adds:

> Abstract theories of personality, heavy emphasis on perceiving overt symptoms, preoccupation with diagnoses and technique combine with a suspicious attitude toward the therapist's own inner promptings to produce an impersonal, mechanical, and detached attitude in the therapist—and soon thereafter in the patient—an attitude which foredooms the whole enterprise. (4)

We can look at painting as another analogy. An experienced painter has certain techniques of color, line, shading, perspective, etc., at her/his disposal. As forms are painted onto the canvas the artist observes it, perhaps from more than one angle, has an impression, and chooses his/her next brush stroke in response to this impression. Then the process starts all over again. This is very similar to the recursive relationship between our "brush strokes" (statements, questions, non-verbal gestures, reflections, silence, etc.) and the client's responses (often non-verbal). This requires a "not-knowing" stance and an ability to pivot in the moment in response to something new and unexpected. After experiencing this you'll realize how horribly this process breaks down when the subjectivity of the therapist is fixed in the clinical vocabulary.

As artists therapists strive to understand and articulate their understanding of the client and then to read the client's response, and then adjust accordingly. I often call this endless feedback loop *becoming one* with the client, entering the space of the in between, or the creation of intersubjectivity. The resonance between tuning forks is an apt metaphor for the resonance between human beings in intersubjective space. It is highly dynamic and requires great presence, empathy, and authenticity on the therapist's part. The power is in the now.[1]

As an art form the focus needs to be on a here-and-now connection with the client, an experimental mindset, and a flexibility of interpretation and responsiveness. Furthermore, the foundation of the therapeutic relationship is the privileging of client choice. As Peggy Natiello began her chapter "An Argument for Client Self-Determination" in *The Psychotherapy of Carl Rogers* (1996):

> The therapist's commitment to the self-determination of the client is the outstanding feature of client-centered therapy. Rogers (1977) described this commitment as:
>
> a conscious renunciation and avoidance by the therapist of all control over, or decision-making for, the client. It is the facilitation of self-ownership by the client and the strategies by which this can be achieved; the placing of the locus of decision-making and the responsibility for the effects of these decisions. It is politically centered in the client. (14)

The end result is a collaborative venture which privileges client choice and his/her right to experiment with different perspectives and strategies. Neither therapist nor client *really* know what the best way forward is; and, furthermore, the end results of a strategy, whether it produced the desired result or not, will always provide new data with which to fit into the next dialogue and experimental action. In the maze of life the point is to learn from the dead ends not necessarily to avoid them in the first place; therapists are like catalysts, simply making the learning process more efficient. The therapist's stubborn insistence on the "right," "prudent," or "rational" course of action (or silently resentful acquiescence to the client's choice) is once again the *battle of wills* at the expense of intersubjectivity and the relationship. Life experience is the best teacher.

The engagement and artistry of the therapeutic relationship translates into the engagement and art of living.

The focus in training mental health professionals needs to change from theory to practice. In particular, training should focus on dialogic skill and a pragmatic perspective that supports dialogue, relationship, authenticity, intimacy, presence, non-judgmentalness, subject-to-subject (versus hierarchical) relating, intersubjectivity, flexibility of responsiveness, and a developmental perspective (in other words, all psychological difficulties are developmental difficulties).

THE ROGERIAN STANCE AND PERSPECTIVE

Though I can't seem to stop referencing him and his work, I'm not advocating a return to client-centered therapy as practiced by Carl Rogers. To the degree that we have transformed our own nature we can use our embodied human wisdom to authentically and collaboratively relanguage, reinterpret, or redescribe our client's experience. Carl Rogers's work stands as an exemplar of intersubjectivity and for this we are forever indebted. For those interested in complete transcripts, Carl Rogers's own reflections on his work, and insightful commentary I recommend *The Psychotherapy of Carl Rogers* (1996).

Rogers was also clear that his effectiveness as a psychotherapist was crucially dependent on his own personal growth or transformation—or as we would say it, on the character of his subjectivity. As he put it in *On Becoming a Person: A Therapist's View of Psychotherapy* (1961):

> The degree to which I can create relationships, which facilitate the growth of others as separate persons, is a measure of the growth I have achieved in myself. (56)

Presciently, he saw how the therapeutic relationship (intersubjectivity) was the bridge between his transformation and his client's.

The point is intersubjectivity, and Rogers described its conditions, performed it, and embodied it. The coalescence of unconditional positive regard, accurate empathy, and therapist congruence (authenticity) constitute a stance, perspective, and practice critical to the creation and maintenance of intersubjective space. Intersubjectivity is the center of gravity. However, it is the integration of intersubjectivity and redescription where the magic happens!

In my article "Practical Applications of the Rogerian Perspective in Postmodern Therapy" (2001) I maintained that Carl Rogers out-postmoderned the postmodernists, at least in his relationship with the client. Yet, as mentioned before, Carl Rogers, like so many master therapists, was unable to make the final breach into the language paradigm.

RECONTEXTUALIZING "WHAT WORKS" IN MENTAL HEALTH

Many mental health professionals have skillsets that they could utilize and greatly expand if they could lose the theoretical and categorical lenses that limit their receptivity, flexibility, and responsiveness thus preventing them from entering and staying in intersubjective space.

Fear not mental health professionals! The pragmatic spirit of mental health has been forging ahead despite the drag and weight of its unnecessary and harmful assumptions. Pills, mindfulness, Socratic inquiry, assertiveness training, empathy, contextualizing childhood formative experiences, behavioral experiments—and on and on—are all wonderful tools! We can stop performing the practices that script people as (passive, dependent, incompetent, helpless, and insecure) patients with diagnoses, and instead position them as experts in their own lives, responsible for their own lives and actions. Without the distinction of "mental illness" we're all on the path of personal growth—*interdependent* on one another.

Having gotten rid of the classifying word game, as helpers we can spend much more time developing the interpersonal and dialogic skill necessary to facilitate personal growth. Instead of getting good at diagnosing "borderline personality disorder" we can become skilled in connection, compassion, collaboration, conflict resolution, explanation, persuasion, privileging client choice, integrating human wisdom, and the use of all the already existing professional tools—all of which are crucial for maintaining and nurturing helping relationships.

The language of empowerment or wellness includes all of the perspectives, concepts, and strategies that are available—to all of us on the path toward personal growth—in books and seminars. The personal growth industry is vast and to enumerate it would be impractical and beyond the scope of this chapter. The important thing to recognize is that personal and spiritual growth (aka human transformation) is for everyone. We're all in the same subjective dilemma. We're all on the journey to develop greater competence and to acquire a lifestyle that discovers, develops, and maintains wellness, a subjective sense of well-being, and purpose. The integration of personal lived experience with the tools of personal growth—including self-help and wellness—is an art form. Robert Fancher, philosopher, author, psychotherapist, as well as noted critic of the mental health profession, asserts:

> Mental health care exerts an influence on the basis of its claim to scientific status, but that claim is false. What it actually does is induct people into understanding life in certain ways that are artifacts of the cultures of healing. (1997, 4)

The psychotherapist as artist is a liaison between collective human wisdom and the client's frame of reference. Such a *conduit* function requires a heightened sensitivity, authenticity, non-judgmentalness, empathy, receptiveness, flexibility, responsiveness, timing, assertiveness yet openness, and a particular comfort with intimacy, uncertainty, ambiguity, and ambivalence.

Let's start with what the mental health profession already has going for it; with one very important caveat—you have to take the skills and strategies out of their pathologizing and deficit-based context. What you're left with are tools to help people feel better, have more satisfying relationships, accomplish their objectives, and have more meaningful lives. To illustrate what I mean I'll use two examples of well-known strategies.

Marsha Linehan's dialectical behavior therapy (1993) is filled with practical strategies for people to deal with their emotional reactivity and impulsiveness. Mindfulness, distress tolerance strategies, radical acceptance, interpersonal skills, and chain analysis are among the brilliant strategies to help people deal with overwhelming emotions and behavioral problems. Yet the fundamental premise of her work is based on the *abstraction* of "borderline personality disorder." Like all the DSM (Diagnostic and Statistical Manual) diagnoses just because so-called "symptoms" tend to cluster together doesn't imply a physical-neuronal-chemical entity inside the person—a "disorder"—unilaterally causing these "symptoms."

Human behavior and subjective experience always have neural correlates; but with neuroplasticity and complexity theory we take full advantage of the way thinking, language, and behavior (including environment and lifestyle) change neuronal patterns. So changes in our thinking and behavior have neural correlates as well. Causality goes both ways; the brain and behavior/thinking are reflexively related. The observed consistency of any "diagnosis" or cluster of behaviors over time is only due to etched neuronal circuits that are both cause and effect of long-entrenched habits and patterns of being; not to mention its persistence resulting from the reifying effect of labeling. And, of course, all this is further cemented into place by the "patient" identity (narratively supported) and the pathologizing systemic complementarity (i.e., the way significant others treat the person as "broken," "fragile," less than competent, unrealistic, "mentally ill," "bipolar," etc.).

When you posit someone having a "borderline personality disorder" you've set up a conceptual framework or lens for that person and all their "clinical" helpers to interpret all that person's difficulties. Yes, the language perpetuates in a self-fulfilling fashion the very emotional, cognitive, and behavioral problems it purportedly is there the help with. Because mental health professionals have reified the category "borderline personality disorder" as an illness or physical condition, they are woefully inept in dealing with (1) the subjectivity at the core of the behavior and (2) the disruptive behavior that often interferes with intersubjectivity. This explains the negative feelings and connotations (i.e., resentment and helplessness) that go with this label. If you don't posit a "condition" then you have to learn to productively engage both subjectivity and behavior. As a therapist from this postmodern coaching perspective your interpersonal skills as well as the range of clients you are able to work with are forever growing and expanding.

Numerous other modalities (cognitive behavioral therapy, interpersonal psychotherapy, mindfulness, motivational interviewing, etc.) are filled with wonderful practical strategies. Yet, at the same time, the debilitating context—represented by the use of pathologizing or clinical words—is largely invisible. It is as if the struggling *pragmatic spirit* of mental health has been sabotaged by the ideology of its misbegotten assumptions.

Mary Ellen Copeland's WRAP program while wellness focused and on the whole sensitive to language and striving toward neuroplasticity is still bound to the medical/pathological model by its frequent and foundational use of the term "symptoms." Note in the introduction on the WRAP website the masterful eschewing of clinical language:

> The Wellness Recovery Action Plan®, or WRAP®, is an evidence-based system that is used world-wide by people who are dealing with mental health and other kinds of health challenges, and by people who want to attain the highest possible level of wellness. It was developed by a group of people who have a lived experience of mental health difficulties; people who were searching for ways to resolve issues that had been troubling them for a long time. WRAP® involves listing your personal resources, your Wellness Tools, and then using those resources to develop Action Plans to use in specific situations which are determined by you. WRAP® is adaptable to any situation. WRAP® also includes a Crisis Plan or Advance Directive. (Copeland, 2013)

Unfortunately, the WRAP system itself foundationally uses the term "symptoms" which is highly symbolic in designating and invisible condition with one-way causality:

> Make a list of what you need to do in order to keep your symptoms from getting worse. (ibid.)

The languaging of the former Copeland paragraph creates a new reality, a new possibility in line with the purpose of this book. The latter sentence incorporating the phrase "keep your symptoms from getting worse" creates the "patient" and the whole clinical reality all over again, hence the strange modernist-postmodernist chimera so characteristic of this paradigm struggling to emerge.

The term "symptoms" always implies effects of a cause, i.e., a "disease." From the perspective of neuroplasticity what would otherwise be called "symptoms" are referred to as behaviors, feelings, thoughts, experiences, and perceptions; two of which—behaviors and thoughts—can be altered to change the putative "cause." Remember correlation not causation; and correlation means dual causality or reflexivity.

To use the word "symptom" in connection with difficulties with emotions or living is to posit a whole worldview. Symptoms are only surface manifestations of disease, in this case, chemical imbalances or childhood trauma. Symptoms correlate into diagnoses (a nifty word game), which makes the person into a "patient." The patient's illness requires treatment by professionals and before we know it a person has been transformed into a member of a subculture we call "the mentally ill." And, this is not like a chess club—a person's identity is wrapped up in this one. All of this is conventionally and institutionally spoken into existence.

If the WRAP system and DBT were in the self-help section available to everyone as popular self-help books (Don't we all need information and strategies to maintain and enhance our wellness?) you'd never see the phrase "your symptoms." Do Eckhart Tolle, Anthony Robbins, Iyanla Vanzant, Paulo Coelho, Rick Warren, or any other self-help authors talk about "your symptoms"?

The now popular idea of "recovery" is right out of this illness context, and ironically supports it. Recover from what? An illness! In the context of the (unnecessary) illness paradigm recovery strategies, including WRAP, are supplements and palliatives to the *real* issue: the "chemical imbalance." As part of the "recovery" focus mental health professionals have been interested, at least on paper, in client goals. But they still *insist on the means*: compliance with "medications." The metaphysical essence ("chemical imbalance") is alive and well in the recovery culture; it's always in the background and comes to the foreground when one lacks the skill and perspective needed on the playing field of life, resulting in excessive stress or frustration and, if left unaddressed long enough, may lead to a "breakdown" (a beloved term in all cultures).

"Breakdowns" (mental) are often a result of patterns of thinking, feeling, and behavior that escalate without the person recognizing warning signs, say of stress, fearfulness, sadness. Self-knowledge is required. Like knowing the warning signs of a cold we can "nip it in the bud"—same for mental stress. If we don't push through the fears and frustrations that we experience on life's playing field into a new level of performance (perspective and action) then we retreat off the playing field. Now on the sidelines, paralyzed into inaction, escalating self-defeating patterns (of thought, feeling, and behavior) and counterproductive habits can develop (including substance abuse) and feed back on themselves. Our challenging circumstances pile up and get worse as our ability to meet the challenge diminishes, thus making us feel even worse and so on in a *vicious cycle*. Suppressing our disturbing feelings perpetuates them to the point of explosion, uncontrollable crying, hearing things, panic, etc. People love to call this a "breakdown" when, in fact, it is part of the natural cycle of prolonged suppression of feeling/thinking as if they were too dangerous or threatening to examine. Feelings are information, points of view, albeit most often distorted, greatly exaggerated, one-sided—like a house of mirrors. However, we don't see how distorted they are if we don't examine them and put them in perspective—they just appear as truth. The origins of so-called "addictions," so-called "nervous breakdowns," so-called "manic episodes," so-called "panic attacks," so-called "psychotic breaks" and of various counterproductive behaviors in general are patterns of thinking, feeling, and behaving, all of which if intervened upon early enough and consistently enough can be "nipped in the bud." This is true despite whatever degree of "genetic propensity" a person may have for various counterproductive patterns of thinking, feeling, and behavior. Pills *used artfully* interfere far less in the transformative process leading to personal responsibility and self-determination.

Taking this one step further we look to a wellness focus. A big part of life is taking personal responsibility for one's wellnesss—in terms of its maintenance, development, and ongoing enhancement. Spiritual/personal growth or human transformation should be a senior commitment in a person's wellness profile. A focus on wellness and personal growth keeps us focusing in a positive direction as opposed to being anxious over having a mental relapse (as is typical with the disease model)—focus on what you want, not what you don't want!

In a modernist world where "knowledge" and "realities" are *obvious* as well as sources of ego-driven power (aka self-esteem) I expect and accept the strange, unstable, incompatible, and conflicting realities/vocabularies of *pathology* and *empowerment* to coexist for a time. But I also predict that the power and efficacy of the postmodern linguistic paradigm to prevail in due course. Unchained from the clinical categories, the art form that is psychotherapy or coaching is free to develop to its full potential.

THE POWER OF INTIMACY AND IN-THE-MOMENT RECEPTIVITY AND RESPONSIVENESS

Our clients are always manifesting their subjectivity. During the therapy session client and therapist are often separated by social games, pretense, roles, and expectations that obscure for both therapist and client what's happening on a deeper subjective level. Meanwhile, the body is speaking authentically, loud and clear despite the chitchat going on on the surface. However, avoiding the bait of various narrative reenactments, social games, and other relational pulls we hone in on the nuances and subtleties of right brain to right brain communication (attunement) in the service of the client's unfolding subjectivity. This needs to be done artfully so as to avoid becoming a "therapist." Identifying with the role of therapist is a surefire way to sacrifice many of the necessary conditions of intersubjectivity, including a subject-to-subject conversational tone as well as the authenticity of our personhood.

The therapist's in-the-moment authenticity engenders that of the client and the experience is that of real dialogic vulnerability and intimacy. We can stay artfully connected to our clients whether they're reenacting their patterns with us during the therapy session or they're retreating into their heads (as a result of emotional overwhelm) when relating other emotionally charged experiences. We always want to stay fully present in the moment in dialogue with our clients even as they convey very traumatic memories. This is a very active engagement and could be the subject of another book.

The point being that intersubjectivity allows for the client's *here and now experiential recognition* of their subjectivity and patterns of being. It requires an in-the-moment sensitivity, receptivity, and the responsiveness of an improvisational musician.

SUBJECTIVITY AND LANGUAGE AS THE MEDIUM OF THIS ART FORM

Psychology and mental health in general assume that there is a core inner "self" that operates the body. Religious and secular law assume that this "self" is capable of making the "right" or responsible choices, thereby legitimizing free will and the religious and legal consequences for our actions, namely, salvation (or not) and government enforced legal punishment (or not), respectively. The modernist notion of self means that barring a legally defined state of "insanity," the self is capable of choosing right from wrong, and, additionally, is capable of rational or prudent choices.

The postmodernists, having delved more deeply into the human condition from a variety of perspectives (including historical, literary, philosophical, etc.), have come up with a better description—*subjectivity*. The term *subject* denotes an individual instance of or representation of subjectivity. The subject differs from the notion of self by the recognition of social, cultural, and linguistic origins or constitution. Nick Mansfield in his *Subjectivity: Theories of the Self from Freud to Haraway* (2000) elucidates the difference:

> Before proceeding, it is worth dwelling on the word "subject" and its meaning, since it is this term that is most often used in cultural theories about the self. Although the two are sometimes used interchangeably, the word "self" does not capture the sense of social and cultural entanglement that is implicit in the word "subject": the way our immediate daily life is always already caught up in complex political, social, and philosophical—that is, shared concerns. . . . In this way, the subject is always linked to something outside of it—an idea or principle or the society of other subjects. It is this linkage that the word "subject" insists upon. . . . The word subject, therefore, proposes that the self is not a separate and isolated entity, but one that operates at the intersection of general truths and shared principles. It is the nature of these truths and principles, whether they determine or are determined by us as individ-

> uals—in short, the range of their power—that has dominated theory and debate. (3)

Bugental's entire first chapter in the *Art of the Psychotherapist* is devoted to the topic of subjectivity. Because it is the nuances and subtleties of interpersonal dialogue that constitute the matrix of effective psychotherapy and it is this intimacy that is the basis of individual transformation, it is very clear that subjectivity and intersubjectivity are far better terms. They take into consideration the dialogical constitution of the person or subject—we are created in dialogue. Harry Goolishian and Harlene Anderson (Anderson, 1997) called their postmodern therapy work collaborative language systems—an exquisite acknowledgment of how we, as subjects, are products of cultural discourse.

The profundity and implications of subjectivity cannot be overstated. It is our socially constructed and constituted reality. It is the "showing up" that determines our actions, feelings, thoughts, and personal narrative. Bugental in his definition of subjectivity states:

> Subjectivity is that inner, separate, private realm in which we live most genuinely. The furnishings or structures of this realm are our perceptions, thoughts, feelings and emotions, values and preferences, anticipations and apprehensions, fantasies and dreams, and all else that goes on endlessly night and day, waking and sleeping, and so determines what we do in the external world and what we make of what happens to us there. Significantly for psychotherapy, subjectivity is the closer bank on which must be founded the bridge of relationship to others and to the world. To change the metaphor, subjectivity is the seedbed of the concerns which impel us to undertake therapy, and it is the root system of our intentionality, which must be mobilized and focused if our therapeutic quest is to succeed.
>
> Having said all this, I am still missing the key significance of subjectivity. The simple but profound truth is that we are subjects rather than objects, actors not the acted-upon, and this sovereignty is the essence of our subjectivity. Therein lies the ultimate meaning: It is the autonomy of human beings which escapes the cages of objective determinism and which resides in our subjectivity. (7)

By way of critical comment, it is clear that despite the accuracy and poignancy of his description of subjectivity, Bugental falls short in not recognizing subjectivity's social/cultural constitution—that is, subjectivity is intersubjectively constituted. Nor has he leaped into the language paradigm, as is demonstrated with his use of the word "patient" and the absence in his writing of the social construction of the theories, diagnoses, and techniques he so justifiably condemns (in the beginning of this section). Alas, for his amazing contribution, I love him all the same. Like so many brilliant thinkers and practitioners—the likes of which include Carl Rogers, Virginia Satir, Thomas Szasz, R. D. Lang, Carl Whitaker, Allan Schore, Steven Hayes, Daniel Siegel, Bill O'Hanlon, Scott Miller,

Insoo Kim Berg—Bugental pushed the modernist paradigm to its limit in his commitment to producing results. Even for the postmodernists, the postmodern ontology (way of being) is an adventure and effort of a lifetime, whose beginning only starts with the recognition of the truth of its worldview. In the land of the blind the one-eyed man is king.

NOTE

1. An allusion to Eckhart Tolle's *The Power of Now* (1997).

THIRTEEN

If Language Is So Powerful, Then What We Want Is a Powerful Language

Postmodern Coaching

I'm not writing primarily to advocate a particular kind of approach to helping people. I'm here to open up the field, to free it from the ice age of dead metaphors, categorical imperatives (not Kantian meaning), and institutional trance. The profession's medical worldview as objective truth is the problem, not the time-tested dialogic skills and perspectives of its agents (practitioners). I'm not "antipsychiatry." Nor do I believe the mental health profession to be solely an expression of the will to power or social control (Michel Foucault). And, of course, no sensible person could deny that people have serious subjective and performative difficulties (a mistaken criticism based on a misinterpretation of what Thomas Szasz meant by "myth of mental illness"). These critical perspectives form only part of the whole picture which reveals psychotherapy to be a dialogic art form.

The name I give my work is postmodern coaching. It is postmodern in the sense that it historicizes (puts in historical context) and deconstructs (takes away truth status from) the institutional/cultural beliefs that were hitherto seen as obvious and established truths. It also utilizes the power of language to construct descriptions and interpretations that empower people. It is both postmodern and coaching in the sense that it respects the self-determination and choice of the individual and works within their frame of reference, strengths, and temperament to achieve the goals and lifestyles they prefer.

In a general sense, postmodern coaching is the reflexive interplay of intersubjectivity and redescription. Intersubjectivity supports redescription and redescription supports intersubjectivity. We're in essence an interface between the client's world and life story and the world/narrative of humanity in its wisdom. What would Shakespeare have to say about your problem with your boyfriend? I wouldn't ask a client this, but you get my point.

Unlike psychology and traditional forms of life coaching, postmodern coaching is inherently non-normative, it avoids using ideas of what's normal and not normal; instead it focuses on what works and what doesn't work. Furthermore, in coaching there is a collaborative effort between coach and coachee involving an interplay between their expertises.

Postmodern coaching differs from other forms of professional life coaching in the sense that it is not contained within and limited by the prevailing conceptual realities (a postmodern breakthrough); for example, the institutional and conventional truths of psychology, of our political economy, or society in general. Furthermore, it employs a more radical constructivist perspective in its utilization of language and description. Moreover, as a rule, professional life coaching prohibits working with people with "serious psychological problems"; whereas I maintain that the client-driven, collaborative stance of coaching is an essential missing ingredient in today's mental health system.

As I've already mentioned, there are many distinctions (words and concepts) and practices in psychology that have stood the test of time because of their effectiveness in helping people. Human wisdom seems to find a voice even within the negative pressure exerted in the opposite direction by the pathologizing context. We saw earlier how a system for maintaining and enhancing wellness, Wellness Recovery Action Plan (WRAP), something everyone can use, can promote the patient identity and all its baggage. Wellness and recovery in mental health as they stand today are firmly embedded in the disease model.

If we take these efficacious practices out of their pathologizing (disease naming) context what we're left with is the language and practice of supporting individual responsibility and personal or spiritual growth. The postmodern perspective also adds to these practices the non-normative, collaborative relational stance as well as the language paradigm.

One of the advantages of postmodern coaching (PMC) is that it avoids creating the usual resistances typical of the therapies embedded in the clinical model. PMC is fundamentally grounded in helping a person to realize *their vision in life* (or, alternatively, create that vision, then realize it). Typically, the clinical model places the normative judgments of the clinical theories in the foreground and the client's priorities, commitments, concerns, preferences, and resourcefulness in the background. In other words, rather than trying to make people "normal," PMC offers tools that will help them get what they want and realize their vision for life.

Postmodern coaching asserts that life is about committed engagement. When certain circumstances challenge us, such as various developmental transitions (e.g., leaving home, getting married, having children, divorce, reconciling with death) or traumatic events, we sometimes don't have the perspective or skill to deal with them. The childhood narrative template and its corresponding strategies are insufficient for the current circumstance and we feel like a powerless victim. Often what happens is that knowingly or unknowingly people retreat from the playing field of life and develop less than optimal patterns in response to these events (e.g., patterns of avoidance). So the job of the postmodern coach is to help people put their situation and emotions in perspective in such a way that they're empowered to reengage life's playing field, resolve the situation they're in, and eventually find a playing field suited to their talents, interests, passions, and temperament.

Freeing up our mind and senses from the clinical categories means we're free to empathize more accurately with clients and align with their goals, preferences, concerns, and preferred means. We're also more dialogically responsive and connected. We're also empowered to resolve the occasional relationship conflicts, thus providing corrective emotional experiences where needed. Project by project, exploring our interests and testing our abilities, we're able to find a place and purpose in productive society.

Let us now recall the elements of successful psychotherapy: (1) the relational stance of unconditional positive regard, accurate and felt empathy, and therapist congruence/authenticity; (2) the dialogic skill of moment-by-moment presence, receptivity, and responsiveness of the therapist; and (3) interpretive flexibility and range needed to facilitate interpretive resonance or fit. As mentioned before I will often combine (1) and (2) as being the constituent elements of intersubjectivity, leaving us with the stages of postmodern coaching: (1) intersubjectivity and (2) redescription.

In intersubjective space the client is perfect as she or he is. We're not trying to go anywhere, we're just being with. This is the Rogerian nondirective stance that involves the three Rogerian conditions and dialogic skill (1 and 2 above). When we add redescription with the aim of resonance or fit (3 above) we enter more the realm of *doing* and thus are more in the domain of therapeutic alliance.

The foundation of PMC, as mentioned throughout this book, is the dialogic skill and perspective necessary to create the dialogic space (absent judgment, labels, certainty, inauthenticity, or hierarchical relationship) needed for the client's subjectivity to be revealed. It is in the space of intersubjectivity where the collaborative redescription happens. In other words, within the client's frame of reference we are able to experimentally introduce language, metaphors, mindfulness, and human wisdom from the therapist's frame of reference. We read the client's response to our redescription and proceed accordingly in a never-ending recursive and generative loop.

Postmodern coaching, like Carl Rogers's three conditions (accurate empathy, unconditional positive regard, and therapist congruence or authenticity), is a relational stance that establishes an intersubjective environment that facilitates both the unfolding of our client's subjectivity and problem redescription. Intersubjectivity and problem redescription are kind of like two sides of the same coin. One side, intersubjectivity, is a relational stance of unconditional positive regard, accurate empathy, and therapist authenticity in which *the client, exactly as s/he is, is perfect*. No change is sought or desired. This is a reality, a reality we might call the spiritual dimension. Since clients often want to make changes, achieve objectives, feel better, or have a more meaningful life we align with them in this aspect of intersubjective space: redescription.

Problem redescription, the other side of the coin, is where our attunement with our client gives us license to experiment—within the client's frame of reference—with alternative language, metaphor, and interpretation. Too far out of the client's frame disrupts intersubjectivity; too close offers no alternative perspective. The objective being to facilitate movement in the client's preferred direction.

Moreover, no empathetic reflection supporting intersubjective space is ever truly neutral, it is always in some way putting words to our client's subjective space and to do so is to interpret. Leslie Greenberg (1996) in her commentary on a 1962 Rogers recorded therapeutic session describes this creative tension:

> One of the most interesting but least clearly understood aspects of the process of experiential growth concerns the ways in which therapists use language, framing their clients' experience so as to reflect both a growth process, either explicitly in terms of the potential for growth or implicitly in terms of possibility, hope, a struggle toward something, a new process, or the future. This framing of potential, paradoxically, occurs in the context of accepting what is. That is, the therapist does not push the client to be where he or she is not but rather recognizes the moment of the client's desire to change or grow, which is paradoxically an acceptance of where she or he is. (257)

As was mentioned early by Bruce Wampold (2011) and James Bugental (1987) the therapist's redescriptions need to resonate with the client's subjectivity; i.e., not violate intersubjective space. This is the art of psychotherapy. As illustrated in the Greenberg quote above, there is often no real clear distinction between empathy as an expression of total acceptance and redescription as a pull toward potential and possibility.

Also, the proportion of "neutral" empathy to redescriptive empathy varies from client to client and from session to session.

Below I discuss some of the key concepts and practices crucial to the creation of this intersubjective environment.

EMPATHY AS A RESPONSE AND AS AN END IT ITSELF

My article "Practical Applications of the Rogerian Perspective in Postmodern Therapies" (Walker 2001) was born of hundreds of hours of listening to and reading transcripts of therapy sessions conducted by Carl Rogers. It was clear that Rogers had entered a new dimension in the therapeutic relationship. He had entered the intersubjective realm. He did this by his very dynamic moment-to-moment listening and artfully responding; a complete absorption in the dialogue. His I-Thou (Buber and Kaufman, 1970) or subject-to-subject relational stance privileged the person's self-determination, which as I pointed out was definitively postmodern.

We postmodernists know that Rogers didn't have a neutral vantage point. But he clearly understood humanity's subjective dilemma and was therefore authentic in his unconditional positive regard. For every human being, every moment the world "shows up" in a particular way and their actions, feelings, and thoughts are in perfect accord with the way the world is showing up for them. Accurate empathy, unconditional positive regard, and congruence (or authenticity) are all mutually reinforcing.

Empathy as a response is a kind of tuning in with the other person with both feeling and words. It's very dynamic and very creative. We can tell when our empathetic responses are on target by our client's response to them. When they're accurate, the client will experience relief (and an accompanying bodily relaxation) and say something like "yes," or "exactly." A great resource for formulating empathetic responses is included in David Martin's *Counseling and Therapy Skills* (2011).

By staying dialogically responsive in empathy, you avoid the pitfalls of identifying with the client, projecting onto the client, or seeing the client's initial problem description (and its potential consequences) as absolute or objective truth. The listening, imagining, formulating a response, articulating a response, reading the client's response, listening (and so on) keeps you in the present moment and out of your head's tendency to think you know the truth about what a client is saying. This is an existential inquiry based on a profound sense of curiosity. Moreover, the words and metaphors we use to empathetically capture a client's experience undermine the rigid initial problem description; a kind of paradoxical effect, both validating and loosening up. All the work of reinterpretation happens within the client's frame of reference.

To say "we work within the client's frame of reference" is figurative of course. We never really leave our worldview and enter another's. On the other hand, with enough subjective authority we can temporarily suspend our worldview in order to communicate in language our understanding of our client's worldview. Because we are so receptive and responsive to our client's moment-by-moment experience we're far more able to stay in and work within their frame of reference.

Creative tension, yes; yet the experience of this adult-to-adult, subject-to-subject intersubjective space is very intimate, pleasurable, and empowering for both client and therapist. When these relationships are extended in time, corrective emotional experiences abound to the extent of our creative capacity to resolve conflict within the intersubjective space. Once again, this kind of intimate dialogic connection with clients is the basis of what neuroscience, outcome studies, and postmodern psychotherapy are telling us about what works in psychotherapy. This is the basis of my call for a complete overhaul of the training of mental health professionals.

Empathy as an end it itself is a point of view that aligns us with privileging client choice and self-determination. I say this to help practitioners avoid the trap of "empathy as a means." Reading between the lines of the many published manuals of psychotherapy, you quickly notice the emphasis on empathy, validation, acknowledgment, etc., as establishing the foundation for other therapeutic interventions—a kind of necessary evil. Matching and leading from neurolinguistic programing. Seek first to understand, then to be understood (Covey 1989). A subtle form of manipulation. Whether parenting, doing business, reconciling a marriage, or doing psychotherapy—we realize empathy works. However, under these circumstances, therapists are standing on their agenda while performing empathically as a kind of technician. This is empathy as a *means* to something else. The therapist's agenda is like any other vocabularic barrier to intersubjectivity. Imagining empathy as an end in itself, as perhaps Carl Rogers did, will deepen your empathetic connection enough to create intersubjective space.

In intersubjective space we rely on the dialogue to unfold collaboratively; we're in a space of deep curiosity, uncertainty, and unknowing. The mindful therapist will allow ideas, personal biases, and potential "interventions" to fly in and out of her/his head in favor of maintaining the dialogic connection with his/her client. The transition to a broader perspective, useful metaphors, and human wisdom is about fit and timing; it's an art form.

BECOMING ONE IS NOT LOSING ALL BOUNDARIES

The act of imaginatively formulating and assertively articulating an empathetic response along with reading your client's response is all you need to stay separate from your client. Yet paradoxically the experience is one of intimacy. Staying in dialogue and creating intersubjective space is an act of individuality, a very dynamic and active engagement.

When therapists experience what we call "losing boundaries" and identify with their client or are too directive, they are caught up in their own world, not the client's. When therapists sink into a client's despair, anger, or anxiety they are simply making the same mistake that the client is making; that is, mistaking subjective impressions for truth. Mistaking interpretation for the physical reality of events—as if events and circumstances have *inherent* meaning. You know this is happening when you are becoming disturbed in some way and are no longer able to formulate and articulate an empathetic or otherwise relevant response—i.e., when you've lost your voice. Emotions and perceptions are contagious if you mistake interpretation for truth. From a postmodern vantage point we recognize that everything we see, hear, interpret, think, feel, and do has been culturally and linguistically conditioned.

Clients speak as if they're telling us the objective truth, when what they're communicating—always—is an interpretation or description of their circumstances. Recall the Shakespearean/Stoic truth, "There is nothing either good or bad but thinking makes it so." This is not to discount the challenge and subjective experience of very difficult or tragic circumstances. Compassion is our subjective experience when we recognize humanity's subjective dilemma. We know people are trapped in a reality. Yet we all know that we're in a better place to make things better from a more stable subjective platform; and it is from this more stable place that we are able to channel the energy of our disturbing feelings into productive action.

In the existential arena of a psychotherapy session, where we've created the condition of intersubjectivity, sitting across from us is another human being communicating the brain and bodily states that correspond with their patterned subjectivity. This would be the case regardless of the problem. It seems like the problem is the problem, when really the problem is in the rigid narrative template in which all the client's experiences and people are interpreted. We are stimulated to project onto the world a threat or despair then react to that projection—recall that under these circumstances our subjective take on situations is embedded in our default childhood narrative, leaving us feeling victimized and powerless. They used to say the problem that brought a person to therapy is just the *ticket* to addressing the real issue; of course, the professed problem is solved in the process as well.

Daniel Siegel (2012) talks of differentiation and integration both within and between people. The recognition of, embrace of, and detachment from the contents of our inner world (thoughts, feelings, memories, etc.) is recursively related to our unconditional embrace of, compassionate (warm yet detached) experience of, and empathy directed toward another. To use Zen terminology, we have to check our small mind in order to gain access to the big mind *and* the experience of the big mind is crucial to putting the small mind in its place. And, paradoxically, it is from this place that we're in the best position to influence another and hold another accountable.

BEWARE OF THE JUDGMENTAL AND NORMATIVE MIND

"Language uses us" was Martin Heidegger's bold claim used to emphasize how far we are from being independent agents in or authors of our lives. We stand upon a reality whose constructed nature is far from apparent. Far from *embracing* greater objectivity or a more comprehensive perspective, we're more than likely to resist it "tooth and nail." Because the current modernist subjectivity is seen as truth à la Søren Kierkegaard ("Subjectivity is Truth.") the confrontation of our biases, presuppositions, categorical perceptual lenses, and judgments is likely to go down hard. Yet this is the price of freedom and flexibility of perception and interpretation so crucial to our ability to connect, stay connected, and have our responses forward the unfolding of our client's subjectivity.

We're so used to having judgments that we never question the phenomenon of judgmentalness itself. Where did our values and judgments come from anyway? Did we author our judgments or were they imposed on us? The point is we see the world through our judgments and we reflexively—overtly or covertly—impose these judgments on the world. When it comes to intimate relationships we insist on our judgments despite the havoc they wreak; the same being true of the psychotherapeutic relationship. As we've mentioned throughout this book our judgments are simply our cultural agency; they are culture using our body to replicate itself. Culture says what's "normal" and as such judgments are an example of normative discourse.

Of course the psychologistic vocabulary is a normative discourse (societal definitions of what a "normal" human being is, assumed as absolutely/objectively true and good) and as such, like other normative discourses, provides a perceptual filter that among other things conceals the important meanings of our clients. I'd like to be able to suggest we stop using the clinical terminology altogether, but experience has taught me that it is far from this easy. I can spend hours explaining this material to mental health professionals, we join hands and sing kumbaya in paradigmatic agreement and solidarity, only for those professionals the very next day to complain about their "schizoaffective client who is non-compliant." Over the years I've gained a healthy respect for the way in which social discourse is embodied and the challenge that it is to alter this. This book should help. Absent receiving the *direct feedback* that I provide in my classes and trainings—conducted in the manner of language immersion—I suggest in the beginning just noticing how easily psychological and clinical terminology automatically rolls off one's tongue. It's hard to even notice—which is why it needs to be pointed out by someone else. It seems like we're just communicating objective knowledge about someone.

The common retort I get is, "If we don't use these terms, how will we know what we're dealing with?" The answer is, the idea that you're "dealing with" anything comes out of the old paradigm. We want to engage a process, a "being with"—and see what follows. Every engagement is a mystery, a creative exploration, a learning experience, an adventure. This is a source of great professional satisfaction.

THE SEED OF IN-THE-WORLD ENGAGEMENT

We become the touchstone of our client's access to being-in-the-world; we provide a kind of *dialogic satori* (the enlightenment experience in Zen) experience that not only loosens the rigidity of the client's entire frame of reference but also serves as a model for engagement in the world. Simply put, *our* engagement with our client, with the assistance of the self-overcoming power of human wisdom, is the seed for *their* engagement in the world.

The actual human wisdom employed in a redescription is a reflection of the therapist's own transformative experience. The more experience with a transformative vocabulary, the more persuasive power it has. The greater the range of transformative experience, the greater the selection. The integration of the therapist's transformative distinctions with the client's worldview constitutes the art of generative dialogue. The following represents a representative list of the human wisdom I employ in PMC. I also included particular issues or sticking points that come up while introducing this reality to others.

PRIVILEGING CLIENT CHOICE

I purposely placed "privileging client choice" at the head of this section because it is central to maintaining intersubjective space and all the conditions of successful therapy. Unfortunately, it is as elusive as it is important. To privilege a client's choice is to truly recognize them as being responsible for her/his life—as well as being crucial to human-to-human or subject-to-subject relating. In turn, subject-to-subject relating is critical to intersubjective space and the maintenance of expansive empathy, non-judgmental responsiveness, attunement, therapist authenticity, and unconditional positive regard, and vice versa; that is, empathy, non-judgmental responsiveness, etc., create the space of intersubjectivity and subject-to-subject relating.

The normative and judgmental framework most therapists are embedded in results in an unyielding attachment to the therapist's ideas of what is rational, normal, healthy, prudent, or otherwise "appropriate." This results in a battle of wills upon which the client's self-determination and experimental approach to life are sacrificed. As we discussed earlier, beneath the content of the dialogue is the command function of communication. The client is being compelled, in subtle and sometimes not-so-subtle ways to submit to the ideas and ideals of the therapist. The dialogue is forced into the rigid confines of the therapist's agenda. The session becomes a battle of competing cultural discourses. Paternalism is for parenting.

The so-called "recovery" movement in mental health lives more in the *mental health consumer movement* than in the mental health profession. In the profession, cornerstone concepts of "recovery"—self-determination, strength based and client-centeredness—if ever spoken of, live as empty abstractions—a thin film of rhetoric and paperwork layered over a granite mountain of clinical deficit-based reality. Another example of how theory and practice rarely meet: how the abstractions of practice rarely get translated into practice through hard, repetitive work and real-time feedback. What does it mean to privilege client self-determination? What are the relational stance and specific behaviors that support it? What are those that preclude it? Yet the abstractions of psychiatric diagnoses are often obsessed over with minute precision and exhaustive detail. This is clearly the material of satire; where are you Jonathan Swift when we need you?

The conditions of intersubjectivity (above) go a long way toward avoiding this problem. Intersubjectivity is based on subject-to-subject relating where the therapist works within the client's frame of reference. The client's actions always make sense (at least when they're performing the action) from their vantage point. We have to remember that subjectivity looks like reality. Recall Kierkegaard's (1846/1992) famous aphorism: "Truth is subjectivity." Consequently, it's very prudent on the therapist's part to realize the "rock hardness" of many aspects of a client's subjectivity.

Often in the expansiveness of intersubjective space our clients will come up with their own answers, this was an assumption of Rogers's work in the past and some professional coaching perspectives in the present. On the other hand, there are often opportunities to introduce new problem descriptions, metaphors, ideas, and practices—but this is done artfully with respect to the client's responses. The right metaphor for us is that of a waiter.

A good waiter knows his dishes and is interested in comprehending what his customer likes when it comes to making suggestions. He can describe a dish with the language of poetry, often in a very compelling way. Yet, ideally absent personal bias and financial incentive, though persuasive, when all is said and done he privileges your choice in ordering. Then it will be your *experience* with the meal that factors into future ordering decisions. A good waiter, regardless of your prior choices, will be waiting for you with open arms, ready for the next experiment, upon your next visit.

Having firmly established ourselves within our client's frame of reference we're free to introduce with vigor and persuasiveness new inquiries, ideas, new interpretations and new metaphors; but the criterion of value is fit and resonance, i.e., that they are seen by our client as making sense and as relevant tools in addressing their concerns and realizing their objectives. To paraphrase Allan Schore (2012), we don't facilitate spiritual growth and transformation with dry logic and reason (as is the focus with cognitive behavioral therapy) or a seemingly detached stance, but with appeals to emotion and inspiration as well as prudence and long-term consequence. But our client's response to our persuasive efforts tells us where to go next. Interest, hesitancy, "that's nice, but," enthusiasm, engagement, body language, all tell us how a client is responding to us and indicate where we should direct our inquiry. A mindful and unattached background perspective allows us to pivot, let go of any rejection of our proposal, regroup, and reengage.

Sometimes an introduction of a perspective or course of action elicits an oppositional response in our clients; so we want to investigate their reaction to our proposition. All things considered, we leave the ball firmly in their lap and support them in however they choose. Any course of action is experimental and—win, lose, or draw—provides experience and information needed to direct the next course of action. Life is the best teacher of all.

SUBJECT-TO-SUBJECT RELATING: THE ART OF PERSUASION

Treating a person with dignity means treating that person as if they were a dignitary. Yes, treating the most difficult client you have as if s/he were the president of the United States. This is second nature when you understand humanity's subjective dilemma. Every human being ever born represents a product of millions of years of biological evolution and tens of thousands of years of cultural evolution. Every human being ever born is an instance of humanity's struggle to integrate into the social world while being dominated by our animal sexual, aggressive, anxious instincts as well as by patterns of childhood conditioning. Every human being ever born is nature's experiment with language. The phenomenon of subjectivity is such that for every human being, every moment the world "shows up" in a particular way and their actions, feelings, and thoughts are in perfect accord with the way the world is showing up for them. For the psychoanalytically inclined, the term "subjectivity" includes Freud's *perspectives* of "superego" and "ego" (or reality principle)—not as *things* but as linguistic processes. Recalling from our earlier discussion, genetic and early childhood experiences shape us into a personality or character, whose life-determining impact is set by age six—before we're even aware of our selves. From there on out we're on autopilot. As a consequence nobody gets credit for how "good" or how "bad" they are; they didn't author themselves and the foundation for all their decisions and opportunities (their pattern of being) was set prior to age six. Moreover, we also have to take into account disparities in wealth, location, advantage, and opportunity that exist at our birth and throughout our formative years—this also factors into the foundation of our character set before age six. Sorry Sean Hannity.

Consequently, though we may differ in our embodiment of cultural norms, social protocol, self-control, kindness, independence, and otherwise responsible behavior this should not give rise to feelings of superiority or inferiority. Anyone deficient in these areas simply didn't get the needed training (or wasn't constituted to take advantage of the training given), through no fault of their own. The aspect of culture called the human transformation movement—where we as adults actually address and take responsibility for the way in which the world shows up to us—is in its infancy. For sure there's impulse to do so, but by and large it happens haphazardly, inconsistently, and superficially.

From this perspective we relate to other human beings subject-to-subject or adult-to-adult. Of course, this doesn't mean that we would accept any kind of behavior coming our way or fail to hold people accountable; it just means that the context for doing so would be dignity, solidarity, respect, and compassion.

We also mean something else by the term "subject-to-subject relating." Any therapist seriously engaged in personal transformation realizes that we never coast; we've never "made it" and can thus rest on our laurels (and view our clients objectively). In a very real sense when it comes to expanding our subjective space (and thus improving the quality of our lives) we're just as challenged as our clients. The challenges may be different and we may have treaded where our clients are currently struggling, but there is no better place to occupy than the cutting edge of our own personal transformation manifested both personally and professionally. I believe this is a way of being that is in itself very healing to the person we're trying to help. It is a place of great humility, great connection, great intimacy, and great solidarity. I believe that this kind of relating is what is intended in recovery circles when the helper shares his or her journey of personal growth with the helpee.

In the clinical model the client is expected to comply with "treatment" protocols and directives. The term "non-compliance" is the clarion call reverberating throughout the hallways, offices, cubicles, and meeting rooms of the mental health profession. In essence the client is expected to *submit* to the explanation and/or course of action being offered.

However when we treat people as equals and adults—which is, in fact, the reality—we realize that respecting and supporting their self-determination is far more important than that the "right, appropriate, rational, or prudent" course be taken. The analogy of the waiter above helps us keep our egos in check. This is a radical departure from the paradigm of compliance. The point is privileging client choice above all else. The action taken doesn't matter; life will give us feedback with which to evaluate our actions.

Yet this doesn't mean we don't share our point of view or advocate for a particular course of action—and often in a persuasive manner using the tools of reason, prudence, metaphor, etc. We just back off and hone in on our client's response to our pitch. The important part of the "Yes, but" response is the "but." The "but" represents an alternate or opposing point of view that has to be addressed or incorporated.

But keep in mind persuasion and inspiration are doomed from the start if you're not operating from within the client's frame of reference as we've defined it. The matrix of influence is intersubjectivity. Persuasion is a means of helping people reach their goals and address their concerns; thus clients must see our offering as a tool to achieve their objectives.

AIKIDO—THE WAY OF UNIFYING WITH LIFE ENERGY

Before we move on to some of the specific distinctions and perspectives of postmodern coaching, I'd like to summarize its basic operating framework using the analogy of aikido.

As mentioned previously, points of view (ideas, opinions, values, ways of living, etc.) are not neutral things that we manipulate like building blocks. They *own us* (meme-like) and they are involuntarily imposed on the people we come in contact with—this is the mindless process of cultural agency which we also experience as the judgmental mind. This is the subterranean will to power seething underneath polite and "rational" society, including the psychotherapy session. In the psychotherapy session to avoid the clash of wills we look to understand and master the two stages of transformative communication: (1) intersubjectivity and (2) redescription.

Far from abandoning psychology's (or society's) cherished ideals that constitute "healthy" ways of being or "healthy" relationships, we employ them in an artful and timely manner, with a healthy respect for the neuronal basis of character. Postmodern coaching involves the *artful* integration of a person's subjectivity with human wisdom, including humanity's regulative ideals.

Aikido, a martial art defined as the way of unifying with life energy, turns out to be an excellent metaphor for this framework.

Ideals—such as assertiveness, cooperation, empathy, generosity, rationality, courage, prudence, humility, the avoidance of excessiveness (including "addictions")—have to make sense within the client's frame of reference, particularly with reference to her or his motivations, desires, concerns, preferences, and fears. Parenthetically, this is the way in which narrative works; it's a sense-making, a justification of ways of thinking and ways of being. In order for it to take hold, humanity's wisdom needs to make sense within the client's motivational framework.

In aikido when your opponent is attacking you the first thing you do is orient your body so that you're looking in the direction they're looking (empathy), then while holding them you move yourself in the same direction they're moving (aligning), then deflect their energy in a ninety-degree angle (redescription) in such a way that no one gets hurt (compassion). One clue as to how well this is being accomplished is the felt experience of both participants. In intersubjectivity there is the relief and warmth of intimacy and connection. In redescription there is a feeling of enlightenment (including en-lighten-ment, a lightening up). Light bulbs go on and there's an opening for action, committed action.

COMMITMENT VERSUS NEGATIVITY/IMPULSIVITY

A basic concept of PMC is the distinction between commitment (and faith) and our moods or impulses. There's a reason the word commitment is prominently feature in the U.S. Marines. Life is tough and all of us need to live out of the concept of commitment, even better, identify with our commitments—especially the overriding commitment to the quality of our lives.

Commitment is strengthened the more our actions (and projects) forward our commitments. In contrast to our commitment is "negativity" or "impulsivity." To the extent that we *internalize* commitment and *externalize* negativity/impulsivity (that is, lose our identification with it, à la Eckhart Tolle) we are free to choose and act—without the self-fulfilling influence of our overwhelming negative feelings—in addressing our circumstances. We assert or declare our identification with commitment/faith; that people *are* their commitment/faith. This existential act brings into high relief, sharp contrast, the dominating presence of negativity and impulsivity. Impulses or negative thoughts can then be evaluated as to their utility (thus avoiding the "truth trap" as they appear as "true" in the moment we experience them) in light of our commitments. This is the basis of choice. Yet the declaration of and identification with our commitment lasts only as long as we act and speak in accord with it. Commitment is spoken and acted into existence just like psychiatric diagnoses are.

One thing that is characteristic of being *under the influence* of negativity or impulsivity is that we're no longer living in the world on the world's terms. Frustrated with and anxious over our life challenges we *retreat into our head* by way of a victim (childhood-default) narrative that with some people additionally justifies a self-indulgent palliative response to the pain of being dominated by negativity. I'm convinced that the root of so-called "addictions" is negativity. We've long overdosed on negativity before we abuse drugs and alcohol.

What's more is that identifying with your commitment is practical; it really works! Those of us who've had experience identifying with and living out of our commitment will attest that something almost magical happens when you commit. W. H. Murray (1951) states:

> Until one is committed, there is hesitancy, the chance to draw back, always ineffectiveness concerning all acts of initiative and creation. There is one elementary truth, the ignorance of which kills countless ideas and splendid plans; that the moment one definitely commits oneself, then providence moves too. All sorts of things occur to help one that would never otherwise have occurred. A whole stream of events issues from the decision raising in one's favor all manner of unforeseen events, meetings and material assistance which no one could have dreamed would have come their way. I have learned a deep respect for one of Goethe's couplets: "Whatever you can do or dream you can, begin it. Boldness has genius, power and magic in it. Begin it now!" (6–7)

On the other hand, commitment is not something rigidly adhered to no matter what information comes our way. Commitment is a tool, a powerful tool of identification. Yet our actions are always experimental and they reveal to us that which was hitherto unknown. Commitment helps us stay on track and is a "shield" of sorts from the routine and reflexive patterns of negativity and/or impulsiveness that sabotage our experimental efforts. The point being that we want to fully run the experiment in order for it to yield enough data for us to interpret and draw conclusions. This always includes making adjustments to our approaches and strategies in light of new information.

Practically speaking you take on negativity with commitment as follows. Step one: separate the negativity from the situation. You're not your negativity, nor is your negativity true—this is true once you've identified with your commitment. We need negativity like we need a hole in the head. Being relatively free from negativity—even though we may have to wrestle with it from time to time—we're free to address our circumstances. We don't need negativity to deal with our circumstances, far from it. Step two: address your circumstances. Our circumstances have rules and a logic of their own, that's where our attention needs to be—back on the playing field of life. When we have to wrestle with negativity, it's time to recall our commitments and projects and turn to our attention to our to do list. Often we must fight illusions with actions.

ENGAGEMENT IN THE WORLD: THE PLAYING FIELD

The alternative to being in our head is being-in-the-world. Being in the world we struggle with the rules, demands, and people that constitute the terms and conditions of the world. In this reality there are no victims. Recall the victim narrative is an anachronistic interpretation of us in the world created when we were very small in a world populated by big adults; we were powerless and in many cases a real "victim." Absent any other training, our childhood narrative is the default narrative in which we take on the world. The plot and theme are the same, only now we're adults living in an adult world.

Traditional psychology has put great emphasis on interpreting the difficulties of adulthood in terms of those of childhood. The frequent therapeutic response to our adult frustrations is "Does this remind you of anything in your past?" The problem is that we develop a pattern of interpreting our present in terms of our past—this only gets you so far, and often results in "analysis paralysis." Understanding our childhood origins helps in the recognition of our narratively based patterns of being as an adult; but that's as far as it goes—otherwise therapy becomes a never-ending magical mystery tour of reinterpreting our present in terms of our past.

The alternative to this is a dual focus: a mindfulness-based relation to our inner world and an action-based relationship with the outer physical world. Though in a sense we're creating another problem, that of the responsibility for our inner world, in addition to all the challenges of the outer world, it turns out that this dual focus is far more efficient. The addressing of our inner world is an Archimedean[1] leverage point—a point where the ratio of reward to effort is highest. An unattended-to mind is running on the resources available to it, namely, negativity and an outdated narrative interpretation of the world. Daniel Siegel (2011) talks of *mindsight skills* as being essential to gaining mastery of our inner world, including our subjectively felt experience.

Our mindsight skills form the basis of and integrate with our outer-world skills and perspectives. From here on out I will often refer to the "outer world" as the *playing field*. In essence, our mindsight skills are the crucial vehicle to getting us and keeping us on the playing field of life. We use the term "engagement" to describe our way of being in which we're in-the-world; we're engaged in the world on the world's terms. With experience we're clear when we're engaged in the world and when we're not; when we're not it's also clear that job one is to get back to being engaged in the world, to get back in the game. We have to be responsible for getting engaged and maintaining our engagement. With sustained engagement we gain momentum.

Crucial to our engagement in the world is both interest and self-interest. We want to facilitate engagement by exploring and developing our interests while pursing our self-interest in terms of our commitment (in contrast with short-sighted self-interest which sacrifices the long term). So implied here is a responsibility to put ourselves in circumstances and relationships that interest us. It is through our exploration and development of our interests that forms the foundation of our being-in-the-world on the playing field of life.

Thus insight into formative childhood experiences, pattern recognition, and mindfulness skills are all to support us in being and staying on the playing field. In the pursuit of our goals and interests we often find ourselves frustrated and anxious over uncertainty or thwarted ambition. Complaining, blaming, and feeling victimized (or vindictive) are all signs that we've left the playing field. We begin to describe other people and circumstances as negative or otherwise unfair. The judgmental or righteous mind takes us over. What's really happening is that we've been taken over by negativity and that dominating presence of negativity is maintained by our default narrative. We project our negativity onto the world and then respond to that projection. The world and people are not our enemy, our negativity is our enemy. We've retreated from the playing field into our head where it's very painful. Truth be told, we just didn't have the skills and perspective to negotiate that particular aspect of our environment.

Putting the responsibility back where it belongs, on us individually, we regroup and look to see how we could do things differently to get a different result, or get coaching if necessary. Or, alternatively, we may simply be in a playing field in which we don't have the talent, aptitude, or experience required to succeed. So from this perspective we are 100 percent responsible for everything that happens to us in our lives. This is a very powerful position to take.

The journey out of our head—and out of our past—and into-the-world requires two general and simultaneously operating orientations. First, where needed, we need to reinterpret our past from a larger perspective (usually with the help of someone skilled in doing so) in order to come to terms with it. Second, we need to be engaged in the outer world (which is always supported by inner-world mindfulness/mindsight skills) by way of committed action, projects, and obligations, thereby gaining the skills and experience on the playing field needed to realize our vision for our life. In other words, we only temporarily focus on the past in such a way that we can more fully focus on the future. We move from complaint to commitment.

A prime example is the ex-husband/ex-wife scenario. People often talk as if they were victimized by their ex. They can cite all kinds of examples, and as they do so begin to grow fangs as vindictiveness rears its ugly head.

Of course, rarely is one going to be receptive right away to "You know you got yourself into this mess, right?" But, in fact, this is the case. So once again there is the call for artfulness as we move into intersubjective space and align with a person's goals while allowing them some room to complain. But eventually the responsible perspective would include that we were naïve in our choice of mate (i.e., we put ourselves on the wrong playing field) and/or we lacked the skill/perspective in dealing with them (including not being deceived). With regard to past mistakes, we all did the best we could given what we had to work with. Moreover, at the time we got involved with people it seemed like the right thing to do. Give or take, this is the redescription that allows us to move forward.

Simultaneously, while reconciling with the loss of a relationship, we want to build—project by project—aspects of our private life, which may include finding and/or developing our interests. Developing our interests leads us to people with common interests that then serves as a foundation for compatibility. Such committed action, even though we don't feel like it, helps free ourselves from the lingering moods and regrets of the past.

Moreover, from the experimental and artful perspective on living, failure is a valuable source of information. Nothing is wasted.

FAILURE IS INFORMATION

From the perspective of postmodern coaching, success and failure no longer exist; all there is is *information* fed back to us as a result of our experimental committed actions. Carol Dweck in her book *Mindset* (2006) calls this a *learning (or growth) mindset*. This contrasts with what I call a *self-esteem mindset* where our sense of self-esteem is based on our wins and accomplishments, as opposed to what information and skills we've gained in our experimental efforts. Of course, from a self-esteem mindset we're afraid of failure and consequently avoid taking certain actions for fear of failure and what that would mean about us. We're afraid to take risks. In the self-esteem mindset we are terrifyingly concerned with "looking good" (and, conversely, not "looking bad") either in the eyes of others or in our own eyes. Thus we never get the sufficient experience and practice needed to acquire skill and mastery in areas critical to the fulfillment of our interests and passions.

CONSTRUCTIVE LIVING[2]

Eastern wisdom turns out to have a very different relationship with or approach to feelings. Given the challenge that feelings pose, I believe we need as many tools as we can get in addressing them—I believe the tools of *Constructive Living* (Reynolds, 1984) to be essential.

1. We can't control feelings directly with willpower.
2. We want to recognize and accept feelings as they are.
3. Feelings are information.
4. Feelings dissipate with time if we stop restimulating them.
5. Feelings are directly influenced by our behaviors and we have a much greater degree of control over our behavior. We do things that need to be done regardless of how we feel.

One thing to add here is that the "patient" believes that one day when he/she feels better he/she will do things; when the exact opposite is true: do things and you feel better. Recall, the "patient" is an expert at passivity. Needing to "feel like" doing things is a luxury we cannot afford. Feelings are too unreliable. How *we feel* is irrelevant to committed action. Commitment is our overarching feeling that can put all the other transient feelings (and impulses) into perspective. And, of course, all of this takes a lot of practice and coaching.

THE EXISTENTIAL CAVE

Plato was famous for his analogy of the cave; this is an adaptation of the original. Plato claimed that ordinary people experience an illusory reality. Imagine people who were born, lived, and died in a cave; to them the cave and its walls are "the world." The person who ventures out of the cave to see the outside world is like Plato's philosopher who through the employment of reasoning could lift the veil of appearances and observe reality directly—reality for Plato being absolute, perfect, immutable, and eternal.

From the postmodern perspective we are stuck with the world of appearances, or said another way, we cannot escape subjectivity. But we can improve the quality of the appearances as judged by their utility and correspondence with the world of things (or evidence). We can reinterpret or redescribe our condition and circumstances in such a way that we have more subjective and practical authority.

Referring back to Kierkegaard, "Subjectivity is truth." This is the lot of modernist and pre-modernist humankind. The confines of culture appear as reality. For some of us, the frustration and pain of living leads us to seek something outside of our referential frame, outside our "cave." We might recognize our pattern of doing the same thing and expecting different results or we might take heed when our patterns of interpretation and of being are no longer serving us. It is by *doing something different*—in communication or action—that we break out of the cave of our life-world. It is through communication (e.g., reading this book), experiment, and committed action that we get glimpses outside of the straightjacket of our overworked worldview—the feeling, not surprisingly, *is of surprise*. Breaking through our routine subjectivity is akin to climbing a mountain; and in many ways the barrier to doing so is fear.

FEEL THE FEAR AND DO IT ANYWAY

Susan Jeffers's (1987) book *Feel the Fear and Do It Anyway* pretty much sums up what it takes. We don't want to make light of the often-overwhelming experience of fear (or anxiety), but we also don't want to give it the power to circumscribe or direct our life. Nor do we want to fall into the mental health profession's habit of pathologizing fear/anxiety. Fear is evolutionarily derived and culturally channeled; moreover, as we mentioned above, much of the fear we experience resides in the self-esteem mindset and has everything to do with the threat of not "looking good." Thus we can see how fear can inhibit us from experimental living within the learning mindset. This is crucial because fear can keep us from a committed engagement with life, keeping us on the sidelines of life wistfully watching life pass us by.

Though we could brace ourselves and run over hot coals, or do any of a number of transformative processes designed to demonstrate how our mind is the only lid on our life, we can also use our desires as incentive to overcome our fears. So-called "anxiety" (a word embedded in the clinical context) is better referred to as *nervous energy* given to us by nature to take on life on life's terms. It is often the avoidance of risk or "anxiety" that constitutes the barrier to acquiring and mastering the skills and perspectives required to achieve our objectives. So, feel the fear and do it anyway!

PROJECTS

Many mental health organizations are tasked by insurance companies to have documented client goals which are SMART: specific, measurable, achievable, relevant, and time bound. Though this is a laudable attempt at a rational system of goal achievement, we must recall David Hume's admonition, "Reason is the slave of passion." Most people have a very difficult time inserting themselves into a rational grid of goal attainment; the idea of putting one's goals into proper form, including benchmarks, is a daunting task for anyone, and especially someone under the influence of negativity. Though reminding people of their goals and setting benchmarks can sometimes be very useful, SMART goaling as a matter of policy and procedure is more often than not another institutional Procrustean bed in which both client and therapist must fit (if viewed as anything more than a paperwork exercise); another "one size fits all" *procedure,* bereft of creativity and individual sensitivity, inflicted on our clients.

The idea of projects is very different. It starts with our client's frame of reference in terms of identifying actions and projects that will forward their life in the preferred direction. A well-defined goal is not even necessary in the beginning. Any project that a client is drawn to is sufficient to get the ball rolling. We make even smaller steps by committing to particular actions and instituting to-do lists. So what this amounts to is that an item on our to-do list (e.g., clean the bathroom) is tied to a project (e.g., staying organized) which is tied to our commitment to the quality of our life (e.g., satisfying career and relationships). In this example a project of "staying organized" provides for a more satisfying and efficient way of living as well as facilitating all our other goals. In other words, any given item on our to do list is tied to our commitment to the quality of our life. At this level of significance we're much more likely to perform the actions needed to achieve our objectives.

We can make even smaller increments, in solution-focused therapy we call them exceptions: asking about when the problem is less frequent or severe; or ways in which the client is already "on track" toward their desired outcome. The art of living involves sensitivity and discernment; moreover, we need training, practice, and experience in finding clues as to what works or how we're "already on track" because our reductive mind sees all-or-nothing when it comes to solutions thus blinding it to the clues, incremental progress, and creative means that are there but undistinguished (remember the 150 words for snow). In other words, even prior to the initial session the ball is already rolling we just have to highlight this fact and build on it.

The point being that for people struggling with negativity and a lifestyle patterned around submission to negativity, the smaller the steps the better; and the best being pointing out how they're already on track. We never want to underestimate the value of the feeling of satisfaction and increased confidence upon a completion of a targeted action. Like a survivalist building a fire we start with dry and fuzzy material (tinder) then smaller twigs (kindling) then finally pieces of wood (fuelwood). Once the fire is roaring it has great momentum. The idea is to get the engagement process started which results in a better mental state that serves as a vantage point from which other actions, projects, goals, or visions are revealed.

Moreover the choice of projects is based more on the client's immediate circumstances, experience, needs, temperament, concerns, preferences, and interests, therefore they're more able to engage it as opposed to an activity that follows from rationally derived goals and benchmarks.

Examples of projects include improving a relationship, solving a financial problem, finding a career direction, sewing, exercising, dance, art, reading, writing, poetry, school, gardening, cooking, eating healthy, staying busy, cleaning, organizing, photography, dealing with a health concern, singing, improving work performance, finding a place to live, finding a mate, playing basketball, and on and on.

Even if initially we're so identified with negativity that we can't identify any projects in our lives, committed action holds the seeds of future projects. We learn how routine actions (organized into to do lists) and experimental committed action reveal insights and perspective that can eventually coalesce into a project.

We recognize "negativity" and "impulsivity" in light of our projects and commitments thereby giving us power to choose in accord with our projects and commitments. When we act in accord with our commitment (e.g., perform to do lists and projects) we strengthen both our commitment and our identification with commitment thus loosening our identification with negativity and impulsivity. Furthermore, learning to project (verb) we learn to live life boldly without the inhibiting fears of the self-esteem mindset. Finally, our practice with projects finally links what we do on a day-to-day basis to our long-term goals and vision.

The fulfillment of projects often requires us to go outside of our comfort zone. This is where the concept of committed action comes into play. Similar to constructive living, committed action is that which is independent of destabilizing or paralyzing (including slothful or inhibiting) moods. Projects sometime require us to rise to the occasion and get over our impulsive or inhibiting moods. We have to develop the habit of doing (or not doing in the case of impulsiveness) things regardless of how we feel. We get over our momentary feelings not with reason and rationality but with an even greater feeling, that of commitment and/or faith.

In this vocabulary projects are defined as incremental steps toward realizing the commitment to the quality of our lives. This is very different than what might have been our motivation to take action before, such as doing what everyone else is doing.

Commitment is not just for marines and newlyweds. It is a way of life that mobilizes our passions in service of the long term. Importantly, however, our commitment or vision for our life is ethereal and requires much nurturance (especially in the beginning). So like spark, tinder, and kindling are to building a fire, committed actions and projects are to our commitment to the quality of our lives.

Projects are the rungs of the ladder of our self-transcendence as well as the bricks of the building that is our desired life. Every committed action on our to-do list is a breakthrough out of the existential cave of our default subjectivity. Identifying with our commitments through committed action we in effect become different people. This is a new way of being.

Learning to formulate, develop, and complete projects is a skill. In fact, I often use the word "project" as a verb to emphasize that we learn to "project" (pronounced the same way as the noun). We learn to live experimentally with the learning mindset as we "project" (verb). Moreover, projects evolve. Committed action brings new information that may alter the course of our project. In other words, projects evolve and we eventually learn the skill of project development. Project development leads to greater clarity of life vision, meaning, and purpose.

PURPOSE, MEANING, CONTRIBUTION

The Western materialist discourse would have us go where the money is, to hell with who I am, what my talents are, what I'm interested in, etc. We would simply "bite the bullet" and take on the role that will lead us to greater cash flow, and/or greater status, and hope that someday we'll "be somebody."

In contrast, as we develop our projects and steer our lives in accord with the feedback, the end result is finding greater meaning, greater purpose, and greater contribution. Furthermore, finding a place in productive society where we're interested, talented, and otherwise temperamentally disposed we're more likely to be proportionately compensated. *Do What You Love, the Money Will Follow* is a truth and the title of a book by Marsha Sinetar (1989).

Society was an invention of the eighteenth-century French court. With the end of divine right and its attendant absolutism, modern leaders maintained power in the manipulation of public opinion, in other words, in the crevices of our minds. With the help of people like Edward Bernays, as mentioned in chapter 6 on institutional vocabularies, our minds were like "putty in the hands" of the advertisers and propagandists—promulgating what's right, cool, sexy, beautiful, desirable. With a mind so shaped by the powers that be, it's no wonder we pay so little attention to the development of our own unique nature and instead alternately yearn and despair upon the alter of the constructed ideals of a consumer society.

And, of course, the entire psychiatric vocabulary is a product of the Western discourse.

From a historical context the value of the Western discourse of liberal democracy and capitalism is undisputed. More people than ever before in history have a share in prosperity. Gratitude is certainly in order. But, as the 2007 economic crisis has so dramatically highlighted, human greed continues to go unbridled, leading to a reverse of this trend. In the meantime, individually our focus can change toward the authentic realization of ourselves.

PRACTICE

Those of us familiar with neuroplasticity know that to replace old patterns of thought, feeling, and action with new patterns of thoughts, feelings, and action requires much deliberate and repetitive practice. This is true from a neuroscience as well as a commonsense worldly perspective. We all know how practice works in learning a language, instrument, or sport; now we can apply the same principles of practice and incremental progress to our skills in living and being in dialogue with others.

However, we don't have the very malleable brain of children anymore so practice can be a daunting though realizable affair, as any adult who tries to learn to play the piano knows. This is why we have to use every available strategy, resource, and incentive, including coaching, to provide perspective and accountability as well as various reward systems. Moreover, we want to make sure that the projects and skills that we're practicing are integral to the accomplishment of important desires and objectives. When the practice is linked to an important commitment then it's much easier to do. For example, anger is much easier to manage when tied to important personal and professional relationships and corresponding goals, as opposed to when seen as a "treatment plan" objective tied to symptom reduction. No one's vision, purpose, meaning, and passion in life is to get out of the Diagnostic Statistical Manual. Even "the patient" wants to "get better" for the purposes of having a better life.

WE CREATE THE WORLD WE LIVE IN

The world we inhabit has everything to do with how we see people. As we've mentioned previously our childhood narrative when inadequate for the challenge at hand places us in a position of "victim" which results in an invasion of negativity and a resulting withdrawing from the playing field of life and relationships.

With ever-increasing experience and mastery on the playing field of life we find that we do, in fact, train people how to treat us. People have personalities—a product of genetics and early childhood conditioning—that pretty much puts them on autopilot subject to narratively based patterns of being that they themselves hardly recognize, at least in the beginning. From this point of view we can hardly take anything people do personally, even when they intentionally mean to harm us (that too is part of their programming). Kind, mean, caring, humorous, indifferent, responsible, irresponsible, entertaining, impulsive, overcontrolled, hypocritical, morose, passive, manipulative, honest, deceitful, inhibited, generous—whatever the behavior, like we mentioned in the chapter titled "A Postmodern Narrative" (11) it's a pattern of being imprinted on us, not authored by us. Even as an adult when we begin to base our decisions on our experience, how we comprehend our experience and the very ability to learn from that experience was implanted by nature and nurture before we were even aware of ourselves.

Thus on the playing field of life we encounter other players with their own agendas and behavioral reflexes and patterns which may or may not be a help or hindrance to us. This is a Stoic perspective beyond good and evil (or bad). The most we can say about the problematic behavior of some toward others is that it is neither bad nor good but *natural*; natural in the sense that those with aggressive, predatory, or otherwise "anti-social" behaviors simply haven't had sufficient training and therefore are subject to the aggressive instincts that all animals in competition for resources, mates, or survival display.

Different people, because of varying degrees of training they've received, require different degrees of force in terms of limits. Some you simply mention that "they stepped on your toes" and they respectfully back off with no fuss. Others require that we take an assertive stand in order for them to contain their antagonism. For those untrainable or who require skills beyond our ken, we're better off staying away from them. We certainly need to protect ourselves from physical, economic, or emotional harm.

Finally, if we take this process all the way we realize that the world itself is neutral and that the "negativity" and "positivity" are our judgmental mind and that our enemy is not particular people but our own negativity. We then see that we've projected our negativity onto the world and that we feel victimized by these "negative" people. In other words, our negative characterization of others is our own projection; we feel and act in response to this projection, thus it should be of no surprise that our compliance with negativity is filled with self-fulfilling prophecies. Expectations are so powerful that people can't help but fulfill them. From a postmodern standpoint we recognize that we all experience the dilemma of subjectivity, that subjectivity is truth, that our realities are socially constructed, and that hardly anyone is aware of this. We know not what we do.

A very surprising thing happens if we take this all the way out. We find the people in our lives change. Our experience of compassion and love toward others results in them feeling the same way toward us. You can't help but love them and they can't help but love you. We create the world we live in.

I used to declare in my groups: "People are out to help you! And when this isn't obvious it just means they're having a bad day." The Naikan therapy (Reynolds, 1984) view is that we need to cultivate an awareness of how the world supports us. Recalling W. H. Murray (1951):

> There is one elementary truth, the ignorance of which kills countless ideas and splendid plans; that the moment one definitely commits one-

> self, then providence moves too. All sorts of things occur to help one that would never otherwise have occurred. A whole stream of events issues from the decision raising in one's favor all manner of unforeseen events, meetings and material assistance which no one could have dreamed would have come their way. (6–7)

PERSONAL RESPONSIBILITY

One might think that recognizing how free will and choice are highly circumscribed by our default pattern of being (or personality) could lead to irresponsibility; something like "my genetics or conditioned brain made me do it." It is true that this recognition goes a long way toward having compassion for ourselves and others; yet it is only through personal responsibility that we get a full appreciation for this fact of life. Though we can discard ideas of "good" and "bad" people and "good" and "bad" behavior there's no escaping that behavior has both short-term and long-term consequences.

There is a profound shift that occurs when we identify with our commitment versus identifying with our negativity or impulses. Practicing resisting negativity in favor of committed action and projects we actually realize a much greater degree of free will and choice. Eventually with greater mastery on the playing field of life we realize we're not victims and that we have much more power to direct our life than we had previously thought. The game becomes increasingly about more control of our performance on the playing field whose rules reflect, among other things, established norms based on cooperative living and individual responsibility. In other words it is through personal responsibility—that is, *playing by the rules*—that we realize the kind of life we want, *that we become free*. There is no conflict. The age-old dilemma of the individual versus society only exists from a particularly narrow point of view. This is the basis of the ideas of win-win or non-zero-sum games.

For some of us, responsibility has been "burned into us" as children; it's part of our automaticity. For others of us, with the right perspective and repetitive practice we identify with our commitment and thereby learn to play by the rules.

TRANSFORM "DISORDER" INTO PATTERN AND PASSION

In my experience many people seem to need the concept of disease, diagnosis, or disorder in order to address and keep addressing themselves and their lives (as we all should be doing)—similar to the disease model in substance abuse. Of course, this reflects the wrong context and focus to begin with. If there was a profession, such as postmodern coaching, for people to turn to in order to improve their performance on the playing field of life and the quality of their lives in general, we wouldn't have to "pull teeth" to get people to get help, they'd be breaking down our doors. The mental health profession has transformed the wonderful thing that human transformation is into something embarrassing, shameful, degrading, infantilizing, and disempowering. The irony is earthshaking.

Or, if you're a stigma buster, having completely accepted your subjugation to established authority, you're proud to have a "mental illness" and attribute your difficulties to your "chemical imbalance." To reiterate, the problem with being a "patient" is when the going gets tough—which is what is so characteristic of life—we reflexively retreat to the explanation of our "diagnosis" and/or the "chemical imbalance." We retreat from the challenging, anxiety-provoking, stress-inducing situations that are the very opportunity for spiritual growth (recall the Von Durkheim quote in chapter 9, "the dignity of daring") into the putative comfort of our psychiatrist's office. It is at these critical forks in the road where the choice is between personhood and patienthood.

Due to its intransigence, it is tempting to call a *pattern* of thinking, feeling, and behaving (including our response to a negative worldview) a "disease." Unaddressed, neuronal patterns have a life of their own just like a physical "disease" has a life of its own. But once we've redescribed a neuronal pattern as a "disease," we've transferred the locus of responsibility from ourselves to the medical and pharmaceutical professions, and we become a "patient."

Once again, in the new reality of neuroplasticity and epigenetics, propensity (genetic or otherwise) is not destiny. In the clinical world it becomes destiny by virtue of self-fulfilling prophesy and lack of coaching in the domain of spiritual/personal growth. Translate "chemical imbalance" into neuronal patterns and you're back in the game of life, actively taking responsibility for your subjective state and in-the-world performance through coaching, acting, projects, commitment, meaning, passion, and purpose.

IN SEARCH OF EXCITEMENT: OUT-OF-CONTROL BEHAVIOR

Family members despair over out-of-control, so-called "manic" behavior: giving away money, having sex with everyone and their uncle, sleepless nights, out-of-control spending sprees, stealing the family jewels for drugs, brawls at the hair salons, gambling away the family estate, shoplifting, and even the infamous "mental breakdown."

What these all have in common is an *addiction to excitement*. Of course, excitement is not a bad thing. But it too can be abused, especially when it's used to cover up the pain of our submission to negativity. Moreover, excitement is short-lived and turns into its opposite, despair, if we're insufficiently skilled in a learning mindset to develop our projects in light of the information they provide or bounce back from the consequences of our impulsive actions as well as from life's inevitable setbacks in general.

Of course there are all the usual activities that people engage in to experience excitement: sex, gambling, shoplifting, and a variety of dare-devil sports to name a few. However, another way is through the acquisition of fame and this results in everything from fantastic Internet business adventures to looking for one's big break in the entertainment industry. Excitement seeking can be considered *excessive*, like other excessive activities, when it interferes with our other important objectives, which include the quality of our relationships. At this point we're out of control. But how and why do we go from being in control to out of control?

Because psychology posits a single, unified invisible self, it misses the boat on a lot of what it means to be human. Because our current subjectivity is fragmented we often experience conflict or ambivalence often resulting in our being different "selves" in different circumstances. Without the stabilizing ballast of a realistic or long-term point of view (e.g., our commitments) our, for lack of better words, addictive personalities can take on a life of their own to the complete neglect or destruction of the rest of our lives and relationships. Yet does our addictive personality need to "hit bottom" before we get back in control of ourselves and our lives? Maybe not with the right perspective and tools.

Our excessive excitement seeking and out-of-control behavior is the end result of a long sequence of frustrated or anxious attempts to deal with the frustration and pain of life. Like other addictions, the vicious cycle of being dominated by negativity then getting temporary relief from that negativity with the excitement (or other addictive palliatives) results in a shutdown of our normal problem-solving capacity. The cycle goes something like this: domination by negativity, addictive palliative (e.g., excitement), our situation is the same or worse, more domination by negativity, more addictive palliative = shutdown of our subjective and practical problem-solving capacity. Excitement is like a drug that we use at the expense of solving our subjective and practical problems. In general, with prolonged frustration with living, the trajectory for some is hopelessness and immobilization (e.g., feeling depressed), for others it's addictive behavior including hyperactivity in search of excitement/fame (e.g., so-called "mania"). Often both.

Ideally, we simply want to recognize that we're stuck on the playing field of life, separate the negativity from the situation, and experiment with actions and/or perspectives until we get unstuck—and/or get the necessary coaching. However, it doesn't always work this way, especially in the early stages. We may tolerate being stuck and just put up with the negativity. Prolonged submission to negativity (including stress) affects both mind and body and provides plenty of warning signs. So as soon as possible we want to nip this downward spiral in the bud and get back on the playing field.

However, as the old saying goes, "though hard to detect early, easier to intervene; easy to detect later but harder to intervene." The analogy to a cold is apropos. In the early stages of a cold we can "nip it in the bud" with rest, taking it easy, and perhaps some zinc or the like. Later, once having caught the cold, we simply have to ride it out. If we get good at recognizing the early warning signs of a cold (low energy, sinus pressure, headache, etc.) we can avoid getting colds in the first place.

Some of the typical warning signs of a prolonged domination by negativity include difficulty sleeping, irritability, difficulty concentrating, low energy, not wanting to do anything, not wanting to be around people, etc. Excessive behaviors are always a giveaway (excessive eating, shopping, alcohol and drug use, sex, etc.) When it comes to the hyperactivity and excitability track just look at the cravings and the resulting impulsive behaviors—eventually these become alarm signals as we've traversed this path many a time.

With enough experience with getting and staying engaged in life it becomes very clear when we're not engaged; and priority one is to get back in the game. We look for perspectives and skills that will improve our performance. We become very aware of our state and therefore can be responsible for it.

In many ways this reflects the difference between a wellness (or personal growth) focus and an illness focus. As much as I like Maryellen Copeland's idea of returning to wellness through a wellness recovery action plan (WRAP), it's still embedded in the illness model and doesn't add what I call a wellness enhancement plan (WEP). In effect this is what spiritual and person growth is—a continual focus on transcending ourselves, improving our subjective experience and becoming stronger human beings and more competent in realizing our vision in life.

When it comes to excitement about our projects, dreams, and goals we have to develop a taste for the feedback the world gives us. We're often excited in the beginning of a project—I call this the "honeymoon" stage. As we work to turn our vision into reality, the world speaks to us, it gives us information. In all our endeavors there's no escaping dialogue with the world. If you remove the word "failure" from your vocabulary you're left with the word "information." Our map of the territory just keeps getting better. Here is where the correspondence view on truth comes into play (i.e., the correspondence of our ideas about what's in-the-world with what's really in-the-world). The better the map the more likely our success. An exciting vision must be matched with real in-the-world results. Excitement comes easy; feedback (both good and bad), accountability, realism, satisfaction, and peace of mind are acquired tastes.

CREATIVE DIALOGUE AS BOTH SATISFYING AND FULFILLING

Freeing ourselves from the dead metaphors of the clinical model of mental health frees us to engage our clients in collaborative meaning making. It's unpredictable and exciting. Empathetically capturing a client's subjective struggle with language and metaphor is an art form. Offering an alternative languaging in a persuasive yet not subjugating way is also an art form.

Yes, what I'm saying is that this experience is exhilarating and fulfilling! There is a human-to-human intimacy that is nurturing. The play of the dialogue is very satisfying and very transforming. Our absorption in dialogue keeps us in the present moment free to traverse back and forth between ours and the client's frame of reference. This is the power of now.[3] This is far from the "burnout" and frustration which heretofore therapists viewed more or less as a cost of doing business.

A NEW WAY OF BEING

Postmodernism is a worldview, and as such, through repetitive exposure and practice we embody this vocabulary and see the world from this vantage point. Because postmodernism is inherently relational, and therefore responsible, it has a very beneficial effect on our relationships and on the quality of our life in general.

NOTES

1. Archimedes, an ancient Greek inventor, physicist, mathematician, engineer, and astronomer, famously said, "Give me a lever long enough and a fulcrum on which to place it, and I shall move the world."
2. *Constructive Living* by David K. Reynolds (1984).
3. An allusion to Eckhart Tolle's *The Power of Now* (1997).

FOURTEEN

Postmodern Guerilla Tactics in Modernist Institutions

Many a student has had her/his mind blown and reality altered during a weekend postmodern therapy course, only to be slowly assimilated back into the modernist worldview of the institution starting Monday morning. What was life altering Saturday becomes a distant memory the following Friday. The depth, breadth, and profundity with which a person engages the postmodern view varies from learning some handy distinctions and techniques to radically altering one's way of being in the world. A therapist's personal and professional background will determine to what degree s/he embraces this worldview. Superficial applications of postmodern therapy techniques are welcomed in all but the most theoretically pure settings. This chapter is for those practitioners who would like to embrace this postmodern framework beyond a superficial application.

BEING A PIONEER

Breaking through into a new paradigm is both a "blessing and a curse." The more you engage the postmodern framework the more compelling it becomes as a result of how fulfilling and satisfying the work is, as well as its humaneness and effectiveness. On the other hand, the injustice and destructiveness of the modernist clinical view becomes more and more apparent.

Like culture in general, this new worldview is sustained in listening, speaking, and acting. Eventually with enough exposure and practice you enter the new reality and there's no going back. The question then becomes, how do I integrate into the available institutions for the purposes of making a living?

To be sure, people vary in their ability to embody the postmodern worldview and institutions vary in terms of their compatibility with postmodern ideas and practice. Nevertheless, it's probably safe to say that any degree of substantive involvement with the postmodern perspective and practice will require some guerilla tactics in order to thrive in a modernist institution.

I have spent over twenty-five years working in modernist institutions while living, speaking, practicing, and promulgating a postmodern reality. I'm awestruck that I've been able to do it. I wouldn't have traded this experience for anything. Our integration into modernist institutions is an art form in itself. In this chapter I will share many of the strategies and perspectives that have made this possible, but for now I'd like to share an organizing metaphor: the four blind men and the elephant.

The four blind men and the elephant serves as a useful metaphor. Each blind man is touching a different part of the elephant and drawing reasonable conclusions as to what this object is in light of his limited purview. One blind man is touching the large leg of the elephant, claiming it's a tree. Another, the trunk, declaring it a snake. Exploring the massive midsection, another asserts it's a wall. Grasping its large ears, the fourth blind man is convinced it's a fan. Herein lies the rigidity of the interpretations-seen-as-truth characteristic of the modernist world, whether we're talking about politics, economics, or social sciences. A part is mistaken for the whole. This is the reductionism characteristic of the modernist ontology.

In contrast, the postmodern worldview is characterized by its recognition of multiple coexisting points of view. Our linguistically constructed reality consists of multiple, often conflicting perspectives. What you see depends on where you're standing, figuratively speaking.

The medical-clinical interpretation of human behavior and subjective experience is but one point of view, one languaging. We've discussed in earlier chapters the historical origin of this reductive, mechanistic perspective on human beings and the human brain. Postmodernism subsumes (includes) the clinical perspective not as a truth but as a vocabulary and worldview. However, this is not how the modernist human sees it. People that animate the modernist mental health institutions see their perspective as absolute/objective truth. Recall that without sufficient exposure to a larger context the smaller context cannot see itself, and cannot sufficiently evaluate itself. Without a bigger picture the small picture looks comprehensive and obviously true.

With subjectivity on the table like this, we see the irony here. The mental health profession is under the influence of a mass, vocabularically constituted *delusion*; and you will discover how truly disabling *this* "condition" is. And, of course, this "condition" is contagious and all the other associated social systems have been infected: social welfare, child protection agencies, occupational rehabilitation agencies—they all use the same pathologizing vocabulary. What is the first question they ask you before they even know your name? "What is your diagnosis?" Once again, not to be too hard on the mental health profession, mass, vocabularically constituted delusion is the state of all human culture absent an investigation into subjectivity.

Understanding language as a tool and not truth, we are free to use language and metaphor to their maximum benefit.

BEING BILINGUAL

To reiterate, the language of the Diagnostic and Statistical Manual (DSM) and the rest of the clinical language from the standpoint of the modernist human being appear as obvious and objective truth or reality. Why, after all do you think paradigm shifts don't go down so easily? But from our postmodern point of view it's a particular vocabulary from a particularly historically based interpretive framework.

Having lost its truth status, what function could it have? We've already established in chapter 7 on the DSM that the heuristic (practical) value of psychiatric diagnoses come with a big price—reification that has life-/identity-changing consequences. From a postmodern perspective we would call this a language of pathology.

Often we're called upon to document that a person has various emotional/cognitive and performative difficulties. This keeps the money flowing from third-party payors (i.e., insurance reimbursement or various federal and state "disability" programs). This is why I often call it the *language of reimbursement*. So temporarily we use the deficit-based clinical language to do so. Nothing will change in this regard. Disability analysts, disability lawyers, and administrative law judges are all interested in the facts, with specific examples of specific behaviors—all the "psychobabble" means nothing to them. Again specifics are what's important, abstractions are meaningless and destructive at worst, unpersuasive at best.

When the clinical vocabulary is mistaken as identifying truths about persons (i.e., pathology or dysfunction) and is viewed as important in helping people then we refer to this as the *language of pathology*. The language of pathology is seen as objectively true. This is something that can be discarded en masse. When the clinical vocabulary is seen as abstractions useful in communicating information necessary for government benefits or third-party payments then we refer to this as the language of reimbursement. Of course, in this transitional stage, it is a slippery slope from the abstractions of reimbursement (representing behaviors and subjective experiences) to the abstractions of pathology (representing metaphysical causal entities, things, "disease," "illness"). Probably better whenever possible to just stick with purely behavioral descriptions.

The language of postmodern coaching or any methodology that is consistent with the relational principles and practices contained herein I often call a *language of empowerment*.

So, in other words, we want to use the right language (point of view) for a given purpose. Both points of view, reimbursement and empowerment, are valid from the standpoint of a particular purpose, that is, insurance/disability validation and personal growth, respectively. In other words, the "truth" is context dependent.

CAUGHT IN BETWEEN TWO REALITIES

When introduced to the language paradigm or the postmodern perspective in mental health in general, clients may become somewhat disoriented or confused. To say "bipolar disorder" is simply a label attached to certain behaviors and subjective experiences will be to varying degrees unsettling for some clients, especially clients thoroughly inducted through time and repetition into the clinical reality. Patience is in order.

Many times in seeing clients I have to get a read on how much they have been enculturated into the clinical vocabulary. Though I won't hesitate even in the beginning to ask, "What do you mean by the word 'depression?'" I often don't immediately in some wholesale fashion challenge the way in which a client has been medicalized. I will bite my tongue and proceed to deepen our intersubjective engagement. The value of intersubjectivity and redescription soon bestows on me the necessary trust and legitimacy in the client's eyes that I need to do the deconstructive demolition work. Witnessing the joy, the freedom, and the empowerment of clients freed from the clinical world has been a major motivation in the writing of this book.

As the process of deconstruction of the clinical worldview and the construction of the egalitarian empowering worldview involve a language immersion process utilizing force and repetition of the language of empowerment clients may find themselves "unsettled" and to a certain degree "foundationless." The material in this book provides the new context. People generally take well to the general alteration of focus and language from disease to projects, commitments, responsibility, learning mindset, skill development, self-determination, and personal empowerment. However, it's not guaranteed that all clients will be able to make the leap into this new paradigm.

One of the tools of easing this shift in worldviews is to explain that these two realities are really different languages and different points of view and that you can't argue with a died-in-the-wool modernist mental health professional or "patient." The point is to be open to this new way of looking at things and see which vocabulary over time works better for you.

SEPARATE SACRED FROM PROFANE

If your organization requires such forms as "assessments," "treatment plans," or "disability reports" we want to frame things right, right from the start. We want to separate the sacred from the profane. For example, while tasked to do an "assessment" I might say, "We are going to take the next hour filling out this questionnaire because it's a company/state and/or insurance requirement. I'm going to go fast, so if I interrupt you don't take it personally, I just need to collect and input this data. Next time we'll have plenty of time to take our time and discuss what you feel is important for me to hear, including the issues that specifically brought you here." Note how different this is that from the Allan Schore's (2012) example (chapter 2) of a clinician attempting to do both at the same time:

> Schore describes the nature of the implicit and explicit processes in the psychotherapeutic context:
>
> During the treatment, the empathic therapist is consciously, explicitly attending to the patient's verbalizations in order to objectively diagnose and rationalize the patient's dysregulating symptomatology. But she is also listening and interacting at another level, an experience-near subjectively level, one that implicitly processes moment-to-moment socioemotional information at levels beneath awareness (Schore, 2003, 52). (36–37)

In this example the therapist does not distinguish the "sacred" (intersubjectivity) from the "profane" (obtaining a "diagnosis" as required by clinic policy). Of course, the therapist in the above passage doesn't view "diagnosing" as profane. As a result, during the course of the interview the reality of the "diagnosis" and "patient" are being insidiously communicated while this very same therapist is trying to communicate on a right brain to right brain level in intersubjectivity. Pathology has defeated empowerment right from the start. This Schore example alone by itself would serve as a justification for the writing of this book.

INSTITUTIONAL DEMANDS

Like all institutions, mental health agencies put demands on us. Less than perfect supervisors and managers, to varying degrees, impose policies, rules, job descriptions, and a certain minimal standard of client "care" on us. These responsibilities often include things like getting to work on time, having billing and paperwork turned in in a timely manner, minimizing client complaints, and satisfying documentation standards which meet federal, state, professional, and insurance guidelines. My recommendation is to consistently meet these demands, always giving allowance for a learning curve.

The idea here is trust. Employers and colleagues trust us when we conform to certain minimal procedural and policy standards. When it comes to our empowering transactions with our clients the situation is different. Absent a "straightjacket" of an evidence-based protocol, the nature of "psychotherapy" or psychiatry is such that there is a fair amount of leeway as to how to produce a result. Co-therapy is another issue that could perhaps fill another volume. The point is that, in general, people overlook our "idiosyncrasies" when in the balance of things we're meeting their expectations.

MATCH AND LEAD: THE ISSUE OF TRUST

Meeting institutional demands goes a long way toward being able to influence your colleagues. Quality of paperwork is important as well. Because we're facilitating interpretive change (redescription) and behavioral change (new projects and practices) what we do in postmodern coaching can easily and ethically be translated into cognitive behavioral terms (e.g., cognitive restructuring, behavioral experiments).

Again there's a certain agency and institutional conformity that is crucial to the building of trust. I'm sure you're aware this is true in all work settings. Where things get a little sticky is in our speaking.

A certain amount of institutional and interpersonal trust allows us to venture forth in our speaking. Recall that realities live in language; they live in one single word. So there's a lot at stake in how we speak. Furthermore, how much a person embodies the postmodern reality is going to determine even whether or not they recognize the profundity and consequence of the words they use in the first place.

This is further complicated by status anxiety; like good soldiers, we might just fall into line with institutional and professional rhetoric when around our colleagues (even unintentionally!). We could be filled with terror at the idea of being accused of not sounding "professional." Perhaps some discretion is needed in the beginning. Eventually, the results you produce will give you great conviction—enough to take a stand on how you speak regardless of what other professionals may think (or what you think they may think). Recall, the health care profession is increasingly being held accountable for results—regardless of theoretical consistency—so I believe we will prevail.

In the beginning there's a kind of split or inconsistency between our postmodern understanding and our speaking and practice. Starting out people often are able to articulate postmodern concepts and experiment with coaching strategies, yet the postmodern perspective vanishes before our very eyes when they start talking about their "client with bipolar disorder." Unfortunately the full comprehension only comes with coaching and practice. Needless to say, the superficial need precede the profound when it comes to understanding. Yet the degree of profundity of understanding is revealed in the speaking and practice. Note, don't be hard on yourself, all the principles of neuroplasticity apply here as well (e.g., repetitive practice, incremental change).

You can start simple. Will the world come crashing down if you use the word "pills" instead of "medications"? Or if you call the prescriber of these pills a "physician" instead of a "psychiatrist" or "doctor"? "Person" instead of "patient"? "Label" or "mental health code" instead of "diagnosis"? When it comes to shaping or creating realities, as any political or corporate strategist will tell you, the trick is in consistency.

MEETINGS

Whether "clinical" or administrative or some combination of both, meetings provide another unique challenge. Meetings are a powerful arena for realities to be spoken into existence, for discourses and interpretations to compete, for an individual to define or submit to definition.

Fortunately we're in an era where postmodern concepts of social justice, diversity, tolerance, pluralism, cultural sensitivity, and individual self-determination are part of the prevailing cultural and professional discourses. Furthermore, ideas of "recovery" and "wellness" are widespread. Yet, as the saying goes, "easier said than done," but saying it is a prerequisite to doing it. As of this writing, my experience is that these concepts—not having been realized routinely in practice—exist in current institutions as hollow and powerless rhetorical abstractions firmly contextualized in the medical/illness model. Nevertheless, we can reference these principles in explanation of our postmodern views and practices.

Don't be discouraged if your postmodern contributions don't fly in supervision groups or other meetings. There are powerful natural and social forces at work that compel conformity and *group think* in organizations. With training, practice, and experience your voice becomes more authoritative and you'll notice people attracted to what you're saying; these are the source of your network.

BUILD YOUR NETWORK

People vary in their affinity for this material; and those who show interest in what you have to say form the basis of your network. This network is composed of a group of people who are open to this postmodern vantage point and interested in pursuing it further. Building our network involves skills such as gaining a certain degree of mastery of the postmodern coaching perspective, being able to articulate it, observing our colleague's level of engagement and interest in what we have to say, and keeping this reality alive in communication and relationship.

It is a common commitment to human subjective freedom and social justice that bonds us. Like any other social justice movement (e.g., the founding of the United States, or the civil rights movement, gay rights, gender politics) we're bound by our common commitment. In our speaking and actions we forge this vision into a reality.

LEADERSHIP

Mastery of the postmodern perspective in mental health is a double-edged sword. On the one hand, your effectiveness, efficiency, and satisfaction in helping others greatly increases. On the other hand, your tolerance of the clinical worldview and its insensitive practices greatly diminishes. You finally see what's really going on, and it's not a pretty picture. What a dilemma!

There's always the option of being the solitary bilingual artisan whose paperwork reflects the medical interpretation. Yet for those of a particular bent, and for those who are drawn to venture forth into speaking this reality into existence, there is the activist path.

Our integration (or infiltration) is by way of leadership. But how? The same way in which we help our clients. Providing value where it is wanted. Listening very carefully to our colleagues and then helping them with their concerns. Helping them solve their problems. I won many a colleague over by helping them automate their paperwork. This builds trust and relationship.

Another important aspect of collegial relationships is subject-to-subject relating; in other words, don't let your ego direct (corrupt) this process, don't kid yourself into thinking you're better than them or more enlightened than they are. It's very easy to be an unwitting meme machine engaging in the clash of wills, culture, ideas; only to create even more resistance as the opposing camp digs in their heels. Leadership begins and ends with humility.

Representatives of the clinical worldview simply inhabit a reality that their instantiation of culture has led them to. From big bang to earth to birth to one thing after another, and before you know it one is presenting a paper on "The Importance of Endophenotypes in Schizophrenia Research" (Braff, 2015). Our life's (humanity's) trajectory has led us here, theirs there. This is already always true. We wake up to this reality. Moreover, waking up to this reality puts us in a position to be responsible for it.

Liberated from the confines of the modernist clinical categories into the creative world of collaborative meaning making, you'll find yourself discovering very useful distinctions in language—powerful concepts and techniques. Carl Rogers used to say (paraphrasing) that the therapist, as well as the client, should learn from experience and think for her or himself and not be dominated by theory.

Trust, relationship, and providing value are our means to influence. The temptation is to want to teach or inform by way of our judgmental mind. We all know how well this works. If the person we're talking to is engaged in what we're saying then we're on track otherwise; back off and regroup. The other person will teach you how to inform them.

JOB SECURITY

We want to provide enough value to our organization such that they can live with what they see as an unorthodox or unconventional way of speaking about or working with clients. Be on time. Do paperwork as is required. Document what needs to be documented in the way they want it documented. Produce more than the minimal billing. Be a team player. Help out on occasion. Respond to requests in a timely manner.

Being a good "cog" in a reliable and routine way buys you the space to be creative.

EARNING YOUR "HOURS" UNDER A MODERNIST SUPERVISOR

There's no question that this is a most challenging area. Here your supervisor is not likely to tolerate views too outside his/her own. The best solution is to make it your business to get a postmodern (or postmodern friendly) supervisor. Absent this, the rule of thumb is to understand before you seek to be understood. In other words, build trust with your supervisor by taking the time and effort to learn her/his vocabulary, speak his/her language, abide by his/her priorities (often legal or ethical), and perform her/his recommended interventions. It is only after this groundwork has been laid that you have the opening to introduce your point of view.

I'M NOT SAYING "DON'T TAKE YOUR MEDICATIONS"!

To promulgate the idea that "pills are one tool among many" requires a word of caution. Many people are very reluctant to take "medications" to begin with and all they need is a professional's "blessing" in order to not take their "medications" and they're off the hook. I've had many a psychiatrist in my agency tell me, "so and so told me you told him that he didn't have to take medications." Of course, I've never said this. The mantra that I do repeat (and it needs repeating) is that "I'm not *against* taking pills. I'm *for* becoming a stronger human being. I'm for whatever works."

The issue of medications/pills is multifaceted and to some degree unresolved. The main point is that we need the right conceptual frame for the use of psychiatric medications. When we work within a client's frame of reference we privilege our client's choice of both *means and ends*. Typically what happens in "recovery-based" programs is that we work on the client's goals, but the medical model being the framework, we of course insist that "you have to take your medications" in order to reach *your* goals. If all you have is a hammer, everything looks like a nail.

There is a kind of ironic truth to this. Because the other non-psychiatrist mental health professionals are also medication centered and "disabled" by the clinical vocabulary, they haven't taken the responsibility and gotten the training themselves to be effective enough to replace the medications in the first place. When having difficulty with helping a client our tendency, with the profession's blessing, is to refer for medications. The entire profession is medication dependent. So absent powerful therapists with powerful vocabularies, yes, the medication rule applies. Currently, it is in the self-help arena (e.g., Recovery International) where people prudently get off medications.

I envision an artful psychiatry based on a collaborative relationship in which the client is a full partner (fully informed) in the experimental process of finding the best "medications" or discontinuing medications. By its very nature a collaborative relationship has better communication; and isn't communication critical in the psychiatrist's decision-making? In an interview with Jeanie Lerche Davis (2007) for WebMD about "bipolar disorder," Carrie Bearden, PhD, a clinical neuropsychologist and assistant professor of psychiatry at UCLA, asserts:

> "We're really trying to understand what's going on *from the patient's perspective*. . . . The big focus is on developing a more individualized approach—not just prescribing a medication, but listening to the patient's feedback on various medications," she tells WebMD. "It's more of a team effort. *It's such an art,* not just finding the right medication, but finding the right dosage for that person, even using combinations of medications." (my italics added)

The space made for full communication is called intersubjectivity. Moreover, the subject-to-subject respect and dignity conveyed in privileging a client's decision mitigates against the kind of co-dependent (as behavior, not essence) nature that sometimes characterizes these relationships.

Conclusion

I have repeated my ideas and conclusions throughout this book *ad nauseum*. Out of mercy for the reader, and perhaps myself, I'd like to use this section more for concluding remarks or an epilogue of sorts.

Once again I would like to apologize if I've offended anyone. I'm clear that what I'm saying is an attempt to criticize and therefore improve upon a particular aspect of cultural evolution of which we each individually instantiate. We're all doing the best we can given what we have been given to work with. I'm no exception. And I welcome criticism and collaboration myself.

Among so many other things I hope the reader takes away with her or him a real appreciation for the implicit or contextual communication that's happening beneath the content of what's being said and written about in the mental health profession. It is here where life-altering assumptions, presuppositions, role positioning, hierarchical positioning, and defining of identities is occurring.

I had not designed my career as protégé of Carl Rogers; but my postmodern, neuroscience, and outcome investigations inevitably led back to him. I wasn't familiar with Thomas Szasz's work until the writing of this book. Perhaps the word "myth" was too loaded; "social construction" may have worked better for him.

Throughout the book I've used coaching and psychotherapy synonymously. I suppose which word eventually prevails will have everything to do with whether or not the mental health profession can get its act together or not. In the meantime, I'm not holding my breath, so I continue, in practice, to refer to my work as coaching, or more specifically postmodern coaching.

Furthermore, I believe that coaching is for all. Contrary to psychotherapy, coaching—at least ideally—is based in subject-to-subject relating, respecting the other person's self-determination, and in helping the other person think for her/himself. Coaching has none of the pathologizing foundational assumptions that psychotherapy has. Ultimately, we're all on the path of human transformation and coaching is a facilitation of this. Moreover, it's clear to me that professional coaches need training in intersubjectivity and redescription as much as therapists do. There may be no stopping the melding of these two frameworks into one profession.

There are many indications that we are entering into a neoromantic age—far from a historical retread, but infused with postmodernism, neopragmatism, and neuroscience. The significance of feeling, subjectivity, sensitivity, commitment, imagination, creativity, individuality, authenticity, and unconventionality is coming to the fore only in a new light. Moreover, with the aid of complexity neuroscience, science has realized its limitations when it comes to human behavior and the human spirit, thus allowing us to avoid its misuses (scientism) and in the process vastly deepening our understanding of subjectivity and intersubjectivity.

To say history repeats itself is to not recognize the incremental change of cultural evolution. To the more discerning, history repeats itself like a spiraling staircase repeats itself. To say "there's nothing new under the sun" is to be oblivious to the power of language. The postmodern worldview and language paradigm—especially in their embodiment—are definitely "new under the sun."

Epigenetics and neuroplasticity demonstrate how flexible and changeable both the expression of our genes is as well as the wiring of the brain, respectively. We are inextricably connected to our environment so much so that it determines our genetic expression and the neural networks in the brain. Causality is two-way both in terms of the expression of our DNA and in lower level neuronal processes and patterns—both influence and are influenced by higher level phenomena.

The question of neuroplasticity is settled. The question now is how do we best take advantage of this fact. What vocabulary, perspective, and practices will most leverage neuroplasticity's potential for alleviating needless human suffering? I believe this book has addressed that question.

From the standpoint of postmodernism, it's clear that the mental health profession has reached a tipping point and a ceiling that can only be breeched through postmodernism and the language paradigm. Its language is of pathology and reduction—as if with enough research and analysis we will solve the riddle of being human with reason, rationality, and the scientific method.

Subjectivity and its profound consequences are revealed as much in the tone as in the content of writing and speaking. If I had my preference this book would be the last "academic" book on the subject. An academic tone may be good for sleeping, but not for engaging and inspiring. In general, the writing in this profession suffers from being "academic": not of practical relevance; of only theoretical interest (*New Oxford American English Dictionary*, 2011); having little practical use or value, as by being overly detailed, unengaging, or theoretical (*American Heritage Dictionary*, 2011). In the new era of healthcare reform and accountability the profession and academia can no longer afford to avoid prioritizing and organizing its efforts around producing success in action.

When it comes to mental health, academic writing perpetuates the modernist quixotic quest for an ultimate truth that will set us free; when the truth has always been right in front of us: through language and repetitive practice we do change. Moreover the elitist postmodernist languaging (quite an irony in itself) in the available literature needs to be simplified so that all can share in its enlightenment.

Language is the medium of our transformation which is based in neuroplasticity. Heretofore, it has been used recklessly and at great human cost.

A decade or so ago I was visiting my ex-wife's sister's church in Syracuse, New York (coincidentally the university of which Thomas Szasz was professor of psychiatry for over three decades), when the preacher singled me out, not because I was the only white person in an all-black church, but because he predicted that I would write this book. He brought my ex-wife, granddaughter, and me in front of the congregation and prophesized that I would write a book on coaching that would touch many lives. At the time a book was barely gestating in my mind, and would continue to do so for years to come. I want to express my appreciation to him (I don't recall his name or the name of the church) as he turned out to be right.

I'd like to end with two quotes from my (2006) article,[1] one from the beginning the other from the end:

> [Beginning]
> Words, like the chisel of the carver, can create what never existed before rather than simply describe what already exists. As a man speaks, not only is the thing which he is declaring coming into existence, but also the man himself. —Martin Heidegger
>
> The metal restraining chains are gone—now it is time for those "invisible chains" to go: WORDS. The vocabularies of the medical and psychological models with their disease terminology and deficit-focus have got to go. It is about time that the mental health profession enters into the light of the broader historical and philosophical revolution of postmodernism and its consequent linguistic paradigm. In this light we will finally recognize that words are much more powerful when used as "tools" to facilitate change and connection as opposed to when used to try to describe some "objective reality" (such as a psychiatric diagnosis).
>
> [End]
> Finally free from the chains of the medical and psychological vocabularies, many people would immediately fit into society with a little extra help. Others would blend in immediately into artist studios, universities, and musician & literary communities. 19th century Paris was

> the mecca for such creative people. Bohemian was the term for the artists and intellectuals that didn't "fit in." Avant-garde referred to those who didn't "fit in" and led the rest of us. Something to think about.

I appreciate the effort you, the reader, have put into reading this book. I identify with my thinking as well as my commitment, so in a very real way you now know me very well. It's been a pleasure.

Fin.

NOTE

1. Walker, Michael. 2006. The Social Construction of Mental Illness and its Implications for the Recovery Model. International Journal of Psychosocial Rehabilitation. 10 (1): 71–87.

Bibliography

Allen, Graham and Iain Duncan Smith. 2010. "Early Intervention: Good Parents, Great Kids, Better Citizens." London: The Center for Social Justice.

American Heritage Dictionary of the English Language, (5th ed.). 2011. New York: Houghton Mifflin Harcourt Publishing Company.

American Psychiatric Association. 1952–2013. *Diagnostic and Statistical Manual of Mental Disorders: DSM-I,II,III,IV,IV-TR, 5.* Washington, DC: American Psychiatric Association.

American Psychological Association. 2006. "Evidence Based Practice in Psychology: APA Presidential Task Force on Evidence-Based Practice." *The American Psychologist* 61, no. 4: 271–85.

Anderson, Harlene. 1997. *Conversation, Language, and Possibilities: A Postmodern Approach to Therapy.* New York: Basic Books.

Austin, J., J. Urmson, and G. Warnock. 2013. "Performative Utterances." In *Philosophical Papers* (3rd ed.). New York: Oxford Press. Electronic Edition.

Bach-y-Rita, Paul. 1980. "Brain Plasticity as a Basis for Therapeutic Procedures." In *Recovery of Function: Theoretical Considerations for Brain Injury Rehabilitation,* edited by Paul Bach-y-Rita. Vienna: Hans Huber.

Bassett, Danielle and Michael Gazzaniga. 2011. "Understanding Complexity in the Human Brain." *Trends in Cognitive Sciences* 15: 200–10.

Baumeister, Alan and Jennifer Francis. 2002. "Historical Development of the Dopamine Hypothesis of Schizophrenia." *Journal of the History of the Neurosciences* 11, no. 3: 265–77.

Begley, Sharon. 2007. *Train Your Mind, Change Your Brain.* New York: Ballantine Books.

Berger, Peter and Thomas Luckmann. 1966. *The Social Construction of Reality.* New York: Doubleday.

Blackmore, Susan. 1999. *The Meme Machine.* Oxford: Oxford University Press.

Blackstone, Amy. 2012. *Principles of Sociological Inquiry: Qualitative and Quantitative Methods, v. 1.0.* Flat World Education, Inc. catalog.flatworldknowledge.com/bookhub/reader/3585?e=blackstone_1.0-ch02_s03#blackstone_1.0-ch00about. Chp. 2, 2.2.

Bordin, E. S. 1979. "The Generalizability of the Psychoanalytic Concept of the Working Alliance." *Psychotherapy* 16: 252–60.

Braff, D. L. 2015. "The Importance of Endophenotypes in Schizophrenia Research." *Schizophrenia Research* 163 no.1–3: 1–8. doi: 10.1016/j.schres.2015.02.007. Epub 2015: Mar 18.

Brodie, Richard. 1996. *Viruses of the Mind.* Carlsbad, CA: Hay House Inc.

Brown, Graham T. and Charles Sherrington. 1912. "On the Instability of a Cortical Point." *Proceedings of the Royal Science Society of London B* 85: 250–77.

Buber, Martin and Walter Kaufman. 1970. *I and Thou.* New York: Touchstone.

Bugental, James F. T. 1987. *The Art of the Psychotherapist: How to Develop the Skills That Take Psychotherapy beyond Science.* New York: W. W. Norton and Company.

Bullard, David. 2015. "Allan Schore on the Science of the Art of Psychotherapy." *Psychotherapy.net.* Accessed August 8, 2015. www.psychotherapy.net/interview/allan-schore-neuroscience-psychotherapy.

Cajal, Santiago Ramon. 1913/1991. *Degeneration and Regeneration of the Nervous System.* New York: Oxford University Press.

Campbell, E. Colin and Thomas M. Campbell II. 2006. *The China Study*. Dallas, TX: BenBella Books.

Caplan, Paula. 1995. *They Say You're Crazy: How the World's Most Powerful Psychiatrists Decide Who's Normal*. New York: Addison Wesley.

Carroll, Lewisl. 2009. *Alice's Adventures in Wonderland; and, Through the Looking-Glass and What Alice Found There*. Edited by Hugh Haughton. New York: Penguin Classics.

Cartreine, James, David Ahern, and Steven Lock. 2010. "A Roadmap to Computer-Based Psychotherapy in the United States." *Harvard Review of Psychiatry*. 18: 80–95.

Cassirer, Ernst. 1963. *The philosophy of symbolic forms*. New Haven: Yale University Press.

Cope, Keven. 1990. *Criteria of Certainty: Truth and Judgment in the English Enlightenment*. Lexington: University Press of Kentucky.

Copeland, M. E. 2013. "WRAP and Recovery Books." Accessed November 16, 2015. www.mentalhealthrecovery.com/.

Cosgrove, Lisa. 2006. "Financial Ties between DSM-IV Panel Members and the Pharmaceutical Industry." *Psychotherapy and Psychosomatics* 75: 154–60.

Covey, Stephen R. 1989. *Seven Habits of Highly Effective People*. New York: Free Press.

Denker, R. 1946. "Results of Treatment of Psycho-neuroses by the General Practitioner. A Follow-up Study of 500 Cases." *N. Y. State J. Med.* 46: 2164–66.

Descartes, René. 1637/1998. *Discourse on Method; and: Meditations on First Philosophy*. Edited by Donald A. Cress. Indianapolis: Hackett Pub.

Deutsch, Bob. 2013. "The 'Corporate Creative'—Five Essentials for an Imaginative Business Mind." *Huffington Post*. Last modified January 31, 2014. The Blog. www.huffingtonpost.com/bob-deutsch/the-corporate-creative-fi_b_4343441.html.

Dewey, John. 1922. *Human Nature and Conduct*. New York: Henry Holt and Company.

Duncan, B., S. Miller, B. Wampold, and M. Hubble. 2011. *The Heart and Soul of Change* (2nd ed.). Washington, DC: American Psychological Association. Electronic Edition.

Dweck, Carol. 2006. *Mindset: The New Psychology of Success*. New York: Ballantine Books.

Elias, Norbert. 1978. *The Civilizing Process: The History of Manners*. New York: Urizen Books.

Eliot, George. 1874/2003. *Middlemarch*. New York: Penguin Classics.

Eliot, T. S. 1933. *The Hollowmen*. Gerention T. S. Eliot recording his own poems. Cambridge, MA: Harvard Film Service.

Eliot, T. S. 1970. *T. S. Eliot Reading Four Quartets*. New York: Caedmon.

Elwell, Frank. 2013. *Sociocultural Systems: Principles of Structure and Change*. Edmonton, Canada: Athabasca University Press.

Eriksson, P. S., E. Perfilieva, T. Bjork-Eriksson, A. M. Alborn, C. Nordborg, D. A. Peterson, and F. H.Gage. 1998. "Neurogenesis in the Adult Human Hippocampus." *Nature Medicine* 4: 1313–17.

Etkin, A., C. Pittenger, H. J. Polan, and E. R. Kandel. 2005. "Toward a Neurobiology of Psychotherapy: Basic Science and Clinical Applications." *Journal of Neuropsychiatry and Clinical Neuroscience* 17: 145–58.

Eysenck, Hans. 1952. "The Effects of Psychotherapy: An Evaluation." *Journal of Consulting Psychology* 16: 319–24.

Fancher, Robert. 1997. *Cultures of Healing: Correcting the Image of American Mental Health Care*. London: W. H. Freeman & Company.

Farber, Barry, Deborah Brink, and Patricia Raskin, eds. 1996. *The Psychotherapy of Carl Rogers*. New York: Guilford.

Florida, Richard. 2012. *The Rise of the Creative Class—Revisited*. New York: Basic Books. Electronic Edition.

Foucault, Michel. 1983. "The Subject and Power." In *Michel Foucault: Beyond Structuralism and Hermeneutics*, edited by H. Dreyfus and P. Rabinow, 2nd ed., 208–26. Chicago: University of Chicago Press.

Frances, Allen. 2010. "It's Not Too Late to Save 'Normal.'" *Los Angeles Times*, Mar, 1, Opinion.

Frances, Allen. 2013a. *Saving Normal: An Insider's Revolt against Out-of-Control Psychiatric Diagnosis, DSM-5, Big Pharma, and the Medicalization of Ordinary Life*. New York: William Morrow, Harper Collins. Electronic Edition.

Frances, Allen. 2013b. "The New Crisis of Confidence in Psychiatric Diagnosis." *Annals of Internal Medicine* 159: 221–22.

Freedman, Jill and Gene Combs. 1996. *Narrative Therapy: The Social Construction of Preferred Realities*. New York: Norton.

Freud, Sigmund. 1950. *Totem and Taboo*. London: Routledge & Kegan Paul.

Gallese, V. 2003. "The Manifold Nature of Interpersonal Relations: The Quest for a Common Mechanism." In *The Neuroscience of Social Interaction*, edited by C. D. Frith and D. M. Wolpert, 159–83. New York: Oxford University Press.

Gallese, V., Fadiga, L., Fogassi, L., and Rizzolatti, G. 1996. "Action Recognition in the Premotor Cortex." *Brain*, 119: 593–609.

Gaventa, John. 2003. *Power after Lukes: A Review of the Literature*. www.powercube.net/wp-content/uploads/2009/11/power_after_lukes.pdf.

Geary, James. 2011. *I Is an Other*. New York: HarperCollins Publishers Inc. Electronic Edition.

Gelso, C. and A. Carter. 1994. "Components of the Psychotherapy Relationship: Their Interaction and Unfolding During Treatment." *Journal of Counseling Psychology* 41: 296–306.

Gendlin, Eugene. 1996. *Focusing-Oriented Psychotherapy: A Manual of the Experiential Method*. New York: Guilford Press. Electronic Edition.

Ghaemi, Nassir. 2013. "Requiem for DSM." *Psychiatric Times*. www.psychiatrictimes.com/dsm-5-0/requiem-dsm.

Glass, R. M. 2008. "Psychodynamic Psychotherapy and Research Evidence: Bambi Survives Godzilla?" *The Journal of the American Medical Association*, 300: 1587–89.

Goldman, A., and Sripada, C.S. 2005. "Simulationist Models of Face-based Emotion Recognition." *Cognition* 94: 193–213.

Gould, Elizabeth, McEwen, B. S., Tanapat, P., Galea, L. A. and Fuchs, E. 1997. "Neurogenesis in the Dentate Gyrus of the Adult Tree Shrew is Regulated by Psychosocial Stress and NMDA Receptor Activation." *Journal of Neuroscience* 17: 2492–98.

Gould, Stephen Jay. 1977. *Ontogeny and Phylogeny*. Cambridge, MA: Harvard University Press.

Grencavage, Lisa and John Norcross. 1990. "Where Are the Commonalities Among the Therapeutic Common Factors?" *Professional Psychology: Research and Practice* 21: 372–78.

Grover, S. 2005. "Reification of Psychiatric Diagnoses as Defamatory: Implications for Ethical Clinical Practice." *Ethical Human Psychology and Psychiatry* 7: 77–86.

Gutting, Gary. 2013. "Michel Foucault." *Stanford Encyclopedia of Philosophy* (online). Last modified May 22. plato.stanford.edu/entries/foucault/.

Hayes, Steven. 2012. *Acceptance and Commitment Therapy*, (2nd ed.). New York: Gilford Press.

Hebb, Donald. 1949. *The Organization of Behavior: A Neuropsychological Theory*. New York: Wiley and Sons.

Heidegger, Martin, John Macquarrie, and Edward Robinson. 1927/1962. *Being and Time*. Malden, MA: Blackwell.

Heidegger, Martin. 1959/1971. *On the Way to Language*. Translated by Peter D. Hertz. San Francisco: Harper & Row.

Horvath, Arthur and Symonds, B.D. 1991. "Relation Between Working Alliance and Outcome in Psychotherapy: A Meta-Analysis." *Journal of Counseling Psychology*. 38: 139–49.

Huttenlocher, P. R. 1979. "Synaptic Density in Human Frontal Cortex: Developmental Changes and Effects of Aging." *Brain Research* 163: 195–205.

Hyman, Steven. 2010. "The Diagnosis of Mental Disorders: The Problem of Reification." *Annual Review of Clinical Psychology* 6: 155–79.

Hyman, Steven. 2007. "Can Neuroscience be Integrated into the DSM-V?" *Nature Reviews Neuroscience* 8: 725–32.

Ivey, Allen, M. J. D'Andrea, and M. B. Ivey. 2012. "Neuroscience: The Newest Force in Counseling and Psychotherapy." In Theories of Counseling and Psychotherapy: A Multicultural Perspective, (7th ed.), 49–86. Los Angeles: Sage.

Jackson, Don. 1965. *Communication, Family, and Marriage: Human Communication. Vol. 2.* Palo Alto, CA: Science and Behavior Books.

James, William. 1890. *Principles of Psychology*. New York: Henry Holt and Company.

Jeffers, Susan. 1987. *Feel the Fear—and Do it Anyway*. New York: Ballantine Books.

Kant, Immanuel. 1772/1977. *Prolegomena to Perhaps Any Future Metaphysics*. Indianapolis, IN: Hackett Publishing.

Kaufman, Walter. 1976. *The Portable Nietzsche*. New York: Penguin Books.

Kendell R, Jablensky A. 2003. "Distinguishing between validity and utility of psychiatric diagnoses." *Am. J. Psychiatry* 160: 4–12.

Kierkegaard, Søren, Howard V. Hong, Edna H. Hong, and Søren Kierkegaard. 1846/1992. *Concluding Unscientific Postscript to Philosophical Fragments*. Princeton, NJ: Princeton University Press.

Kirsch, Irving. 2002. "The Emperor's New Drugs." *Prevention and Treatment*. Washington, DC: American Psychological Association.

Konorski, Jerzy. 1948. *Conditioned Reflexes and Neuron Organization*. Cambridge: University Press.

Korteling, Wouter. 2014. "How Reification of DSM Labels Influences Our Identity." *Social Cosmos* 5, 1.

Krell, David Farrel. 1993. *Martin Heidegger: Basic Writings*. San Francisco: Harper Collins.

Kuhn, Thomas. 1962. *The Structure of Scientific Revolutions*. Chicago: University of Chicago Press.

Lacoboni, Marco. 2008. *Mirroring People*. New York: Farrar, Straus, and Giroux.

Lakoff, George and Mark Johnson. 1980. *Metaphors We Live By*. Chicago: University of Chicago Press.

Lambert, Michael, S. L. Garfield, and A. Bergin. 2004. "Overview, Trends, and Future Directions." In *Bergin & Garfield's Handbook of Psychotherapy and Behavior Change* (5th ed.), edited by Michael Lambert, 805–21. New York: Wiley.

Landis, C. 1938. "Statistical Evaluation of Psychotherapeutic Methods." In S. E. Hinsie (Ed.), *Concepts and problems of psychotherapy*. London: Heineman, P. 155–65.

Lashley, Karl. 1923. "Temporal Variation in the Function of the Gyrus Precentralis in Primates." *American Journal of Physiology* 65: 585–602.

Lerche Davis, Jeanie. 2007. "When Bipolar Gets Out of Control." *WebMD* (online). Accessed April 26, 2016. www.webmd.com/bipolar-disorder/features/bipolar-disorder-managing-mania.

Libet B., Wright E. W., Gleason. 1983. "Readiness Potentials Preceding Unrestricted Spontaneous Pre-Planned Voluntary Acts." *Electroencephalographic and Clinical Neurophysiology*. 54: 322–25.

Linehan, Marsha, M. 1993. *Cognitive-Behavioral Treatment of Borderline Personality Disorder*. New York: The Guilford Press.

Lipton, Bruce. 2008. *The Biology of Belief: Unleashing the Power of Consciousness, Matter and Miracles*. Santa Cruz, CA: Mountain of Love Productions.

Logan, Linda. 2013. "The Problem With How We Treat Bipolar Disorder." *The New York Times*, April 26, Magazine.

Ma, Helen and John Teasdale. 2004. "Mindfulness-Based Cognitive Therapy for Depression: Replication and Exploration of Differential Relapse Prevention Effects." *Journal of Consulting and Clinical Psychiatry* 72, 31–40.

Mansfield, Nick. 2000. *Subjectivity: Theories of the Self from Freud to Haraway*. New York: New York University Press.

Martin, David. 2011. *Counseling and Therapy Skills*. Longrove, IL: Waveland Press.

Martin, D. J. J. P. Garske, and M. K. Davis. 2000. "Relation of the Therapeutic Alliance with Outcome and Other Variables: A Meta-Analytic Review." *Journal of Consulting and Clinical Psychology*. 68: 438–50.

Marx, Karl. 1903. *A Contribution to the Critique of Political Economy (2nd ed.)*. Chicago: Charles H. Kerr and Company.

McCarthy, Kevin. 1956. *Invasion of the Body Snatchers*. DVD. Directed by Don Siegl. Released February 5. Film.

McGinn, Colin. 1999. *The Mysterious Flame: Conscious Minds in a Material World*. New York: Basic Books, 18–19.

McGuire, Eleanor, K. Woollett, and H. J. Spiers. 2007. "London Taxi Drivers and Bus Drivers: A Structural MRI and Neuropsychological Analysis." *Hippocampus* 16, 12: 1091–101.

Mead, Shery and Cheryl MacNeil. 2006. "Peer Support: What Makes It Unique?" *International Journal of Psychosocial Rehabilitation* 10, 2: 29–37.

Miller, Scott, M. A. Hubble, D. L. Chow, and J. A. Seidel. 2013. "The Outcome of Psychotherapy: Yesterday, Today, and Tomorrow." *Psychotherapy* 50, 1: 88–97.

Miller, William and Stephen Rollnick. 2002. *Motivational Interviewing*. New York: The Guilford Press.

Moyer, Melinda. 2013. "The Myth of Antioxidants." *Scientific American* 308, 2 (Feb.): 62–67.

Murray, William H. 1951. *The Scottish Himalayan Expedition*. London: J. M. Dent & Sons.

Nave, Christopher. 2010. "On the Contextual Independence of Personality: Teachers' Assessments Predict Directly Observed Behavior after Four Decades." *Social Psychological and Personality Science* 3, 1 (July 8): 1–9.

Natiello, Peggy. 1996. "An Argument for Client Self-Determination." In *The Psychotherapy of Carl Rogers*, eds Barry Farber, Deborah Brink, and Patricia Raskin, 120–1320. New York: The Guilford Press.

New Oxford English Dictionary, Third Edition. 2001. Oxford, UK: Oxford University Press.

Nietzsche, Friedrich Wilhelm, Walter Arnold Kaufmann, and R. J. Hollingdale. 1901/1968. *The Will to Power*. New York: Vintage Books.

Nin, Anaïs. 1961. *Seduction of the Minotaur*. Chicago, IL: The Swallow Press.

Nottebohm, Fernando. 1989. "From bird song to neurogenesis." *Scientific American* 260: 74–79.

Norcross, John. 2011. "The Therapeutic Relationship." In *The Heart and Soul of Change (2nd Ed.)*, edited by Barry Duncan, Scott Miller, Bruce Wampold, and Mark Hubble, loc. 3132. Washington, DC: American Psychological Association. Electronic Edition.

Norcross, John and Michael Lambert. 2005. "The Therapy Relationship." *In Evidence-Based Practices in Mental Health: Debate and Dialogue on the Fundamental Questions* (208–17). Edited by J. C. Norcross, L. E. Beutler, and R. F. Levant. Washington, DC: American Psychological Association.

Nussbaum, Bruce, Robert Berner, and Diane Brady. 2005. "Get Creative!" *Bloomberg Business*. Last modified July 31. Opinion. www.bloomberg.com/bw/stories/2005-07-31/get-creative.

O'Hanlon, William, & Michelle Weiner-Davis. 1989. *In Search of Solutions: A New Direction in Psychotherapy*. New York: W. W. Norton and Company.

Orlinsky, David, M. Ronnestad, and U. Willutzki. 2004. "Fifty Years of Process-Outcome Research: Continuity and Change." In *Bergin and Garfield's Handbook of Psychotherapy and Behavior Change* (5th edition, 307–90). Edited by M. J. Lambert. New York: Wiley.

Piaget, Jean. 1933. "Children's Philosophies." C. Murchison (ed.). *A Handbook of Child Psychology*. 2nd edition. Worcester, MA: Clark University Press.

Pinker, Steven. 1997. *How the Mind Works*. New York: W. W. Norton and Company.

Prochaska, James and Carlo DiClemente. 1983. "Stages and Processes of Self-Change in Smoking: Toward an Integrative Model of Change." *Journal of Consulting and Clinical Psychology* 5: 390–95.

Prochaska, James, Carlo DiClemente, and John Norcross. 1992. "In Search of How People Change: Applications to Addictive Behavior." *American Psychologist* 47: 1102–14.

Reynolds, David K. 1984. *Constructive Living*. Hawaii: University of Hawaii Press.

Robson, David. 2013. "There Really are 50 Eskimo Words for 'Snow.'" www.washingtonpost.com/national/health-science/there-really-are-50-eskimo-words-for-snow/2013/01/14/e0e3f4e0-59a0-11e2-beee-6e38f5215402_story.html. Jan 14 Washington Post. Health and Science.

Rogers, Ben. 2006. "Poetic Uncovering in Heidegger." aporia.byu.edu/pdfs/rogers-poetic_uncovering_in_heidegger.pdf.

Rogers, Carl and Rosalind Dymond. 1954. *Psychotherapy and Personality Change: Co-ordinated Research Studies in the Client-centered Approach*. Chicago: University of Chicago Press.

Rogers, Carl. 1957. "The Necessary and Sufficient Conditions of Therapeutic Personality Change." *Journal of Consulting Psychology*. 21: 95–103.

Rogers, Carl. 1961. *On Becoming a Person: A Therapist's View of Psychotherapy*. New York: Houghton Mifflin Company.

Rogers, Carl. 1977. *Carl Rogers on Personal Power*. New York: Delacorte.

Rorty, Richard. 1982. *The Consequences of Pragmatism*. Minneapolis: University of Minnesota Press.

Rosenbaum, Ruth. 2012. "Psychoanalysis, Psi Phenomena, and Spiritual Space: Common Ground." In *The Oxford Handbook of Psychology and Spirituality*. Edited by Lisa J. Miller, 271–85.

Rosenzweig, Mark R. 2007. "Modification of Brain Circuits through Experience." In *Neural Plasticity and Memory: From Genes to Brain Imaging*, edited by Federico Bermudez-Rattoni, 67–94. Boca Raton, FL: CRC Press, Taylor & Francis Group.

Sadato, N., Pascual-Leone A, Grafman J, Ibañez V, Deiber MP, Dold G, and Hallett M. 1996. "Activation of the Primary Visual Cortex by Braille Reading in Blind Subjects." *Nature* 380: 526–28.

Schildkraut, Joseph. 1965. "The Catecholamine Hypothesis of Affective Disorders: A review of Supporting Evidence."*American Journal of Psychiatry* 122, 5: 509–22.

Schore, Allan. 2003. *Affect Regulation and the Repair of the Self*. New York: Norton.

Schore, Allan. 2006. *Neurobiology and Attachment Theory in Psychotherapy*. Workshop conducted at Mount Sinai Medical Center, New York.

Schore, Allan. 2012. *The Science of the Art of Psychotherapy*. New York: W.W. Norton and Company.

Schore, Allan, and Judith Schore. 2012. "Modern Attachment Theory: The Central Role of Affect Regulation in Development and Treatment." In *The Science of the Art of* Psychotherapy by Allan Schore, 27–50. New York: W. W. Norton and Company.

Schwartz, Jeffery, and Sharon Begley. 2002. *The Mind and the Brain: Neuroplasticity and the Power of Mental Force*. New York: Harper Collins.

Schwartz, Jeffery, P. W. Stoessel, L. R. Baxter, K. M. Martin, M. E. Phelps. 1996. "Systematic Changes in Cerebral Glucose Metabolic Rate After Successful Behavior Modification Treatment of Obsessive-Compulsive Disorder." *Archives of General Psychiatry* 53(2): 109–13.

Shatz, Carla J. 1992. "The Developing Brain." United States: *Scientific American* 267: 60–67.

Siegel, Daniel. 2010. *The Mindful Therapist*. New York: W. W. Norton and Company.

Siegel, Daniel. 2011. *Mindsight: The New Science of Personal Transformation*. New York: Bantam Books.

Siegel, Daniel. 2012. *Pocket Guide to Interpersonal Neurobiology: An Integrative Handbook of the Mind*. New York: W. W. Norton and Company.

Siegel, Daniel. 2014. "Pruning, Myelination, and the Remodeling Adolescent Brain." Posted Feb 04, 2014. www.psychologytoday.com/blog/inspire-rewire/201402/pruning-myelination-and-the-remodeling-adolescent-brain.

Sinatra, Stephen and John Bowden. 2011. *The Great Cholesterol Myth: Why Lowering Your Cholesterol Won't Prevent Heart Disease-and the Statin-Free Plan That Will*. Beverly, MA: Fair Winds Press.

Sinetar, Marsha. 1989. *Do What You Love, the Money Will Follow: Discovering Your Right Livelihood*. New York: Dell Publishing.

Smith, Mary and Gene Glass. 1977. "Meta-analysis of Psychotherapy Outcome Studies. *American Psychologist* 32, 9 (Sep 1977): 752–60.

Spock, Benjamin. 1968. *Baby and Child Care*. 3rd edition. New York: Hawthorn Books.

Sykes Wylie, Mary and Lynn Turner. 2015. "The Attuned Therapist." *Psychotherapy Networker*. www.psychotherapynetworker.org/magazine/recentissues/1261-the-attunded-therapist.

Szasz, Thomas. 1973. *The Second Sin*. New York: Mass Market Paperback.

Szasz, Thomas. 1961. *The Myth of Mental Illness: Foundations of a Theory of Personal Conduct*. New York: Perennial, Harper Collins Publishers.

Taub, Edward, N. E. Miller, T. A. Novack, E. W. Cook III, W. C. Flemming, C. S. Nepomuceno, J. S. Connell, and J. E. Crago. 1993. "Technique to Improve Chronic Motor Deficit after Stroke," *Archives of Physical Medicine and Rehabilitation* 74: 347–54.

Tavris, Carol. 2013. "How Psychiatry Went Crazy." *Wall Street Journal*, May 18, Books.

Teasdale, John, Z. V. Segal, J. M. Williams, V. A. Ridgeway, J. M. Soulsby, M. A. Lau. 2000. "Prevention of Relapse/Recurrence in Major Depression by Mindfulness-Based Cognitive Therapy." *Journal of Consulting and Clinical Psychiatry* 68: 615–23.

Thibodeau, Paul and Lera Boroditsky. 2011. "Metaphors We Think With: The Role of Metaphor in Reasoning." *PLoS ONE 6(2)*: e16782. doi:10.1371/journal.pone.0016782.

Tolle, Eckhart. 1997. *The Power of Now: A Guide to Spiritual Enlightenment*. Novato, California: New World Library.

Tschacher, Wolfgang, Schildt, M. and Sander, K. 2010. "Brain Connectivity in Listening to Affective Stimuli: A Functional Magnetic Resonance Imaging (fMRI) Study and Implications for Psychotherapy." *Psychotherapy Research* 20: 576–88.

U.S. Government Printing Office. 2003. *Achieving the promise: Transforming mental health care in America*.

Veyne, Paul. 1988. *Did the Greeks Believe in Their Myths?: An Essay on the Constitutive Imagination*. Chicago: University of Chicago Press.

Von Durkheim, Karl. 1971. *The Way of Transformation: Daily Life as Spiritual Practice*. Sandpoint, ID: Morning Light Press.

Von Foerster, Heinz. 1984/2006. "On constructing a reality." In P. Watzlawick (Ed.), *The Invented Reality*, 41–61. New York: Norton.

Walker, Michael. 2001. "Practical Applications of the Rogerian Perspective in Postmodern Psychotherapy." *Journal of Systemic Therapies*. 20(2): 41–57.

Walker, Michael. 2006. The Social Construction of Mental Illness and its Implications for the Recovery Model. International Journal of Psychosocial Rehabilitation. 10 (1): 71–87.

Wallace, Michal, and George Dunlop. 2006. *Eliza, Computer Therapist*. Accessed December 8, 2015. www.manifestation.com/neurotoys/eliza.php3.

Walter, John & Jane Peller. 2000. *Recreating Brief Therapy: Preferences and Possibilities*. New York: Norton.

Wampold, Bruce. 2001. *The Great Psychotherapy Debate: Models, Methods and Findings*. Mahwah, NJ: Lawrence Erlbaum, Publishers.

Wampold, Bruce. 2011. "The Research Evidence for the Common Factors Model: A Historically Situated Perspective." In *The Heart and Soul of Change* (2nd Ed.) by Barry Duncan, Scott Miller, Bruce Wampold, and Mark Hubble. Washington, DC: American Psychological Association. Electronic Edition.

Weber, Max. 1905/2001. *The Protestant Ethic and the Spirit of Capitalism*. London: Routledge.

Whitaker, Robert and Lisa Cosgrove. 2015. *Psychiatry Under the Influence: Institutional Corruptions, Social Injury, and Prescriptions for Reform*. New York: Palgrave Macmillan. Electronic Edition.

Whitehead, Alfred North. 1929. *Process and Reality: An Essay in Cosmology*. New York: The Free Press.

Winnicott, Donald. 1975. *Through Pediatrics of Psycho-analysis*. New York: Basic Books.

Wittgenstein, Ludwig. 1922. *Tractatus logico-philosophicus*. London: Routledge & Kegan Paul.

Wolff, Werner and Joseph Precker. 1952. *Success in Psychotherapy*. New York: Grune and Stratton.

World Health Organization. 1992. *International Statistical Classification of Diseases and Related Health Problems*, 10th Revision (ICD-10). Geneva: WHO.

Wright, Robert. 1994. *The Moral Animal*. New York: Vintage Books. Electronic edition.

Zauzmer, Julie. 2013. "Where We Stand: The Class of 2013 Senior Survey." www.thecrimson.com/article/2013/5/28/senior-survey-2013/?page=single.

Index

About the Author

Michael Walker has been a practicing psychologist in Los Angeles, California, in both private and public settings for over twenty-five years. He has trained and lectured on postmodern psychotherapy for over fifteen years. He is author of "Practical Applications of the Rogerian Perspective in Postmodern Psychotherapies" (2001, *Journal of Systemic Therapies*) and "The Social Construction of Mental Illness and its implications for the Recovery Model" (2006, *International Journal of Psychosocial Rehabilitation*).

Lightning Source UK Ltd.
Milton Keynes UK
UKOW03n0803170317
296844UK00011B/140/P

9 781498 524834